Child Psychiatry. for St...

Child Psychiatry for Students

Frederick H. Stone
M.B., Ch.B., F.R.C.P. (Lond.),
F.R.C.P. (Glas.), F.R.C. Psych.
Professor of Child and Adolescent Psychiatry, University of Glasgow,
Head of Department of Child and Family Psychiatry, Royal Hospital
for Sick Children, Glasgow

Cyrille Koupernik M.D.
Médecin-assistant des hôpitaux de Paris, Associate Member of the
Medical College of Paris Hospitals, Ittleson Visiting Lecturer, St.
Louis, Mo.

Foreword by

L. N. J. Kamp, M.D.
Professor of Child Psychiatry,
State University, Utrecht

SECOND EDITION

CHURCHILL LIVINGSTONE
EDINBURGH LONDON AND NEW YORK 1978

CHURCHILL LIVINGSTONE
Medical Division of Longman Group Limited

Distributed in the United States of America by
Longman Inc., 19 West 44th Street, New York, N.Y.
10036 and by associated companies, branches and
representatives throughout the world.

First published 1974
Second Edition 1978

ISBN 0 443 01797 2

British Library Cataloguing in Publication Data

Stone, Frederick Hope
    Child psychiatry for students. – 2nd ed.
    1. Child psychiatry
    I. Title   II. Koupernik, Cyrille
    618.9'28'9   RJ499   78-40331

Printed in Hong Kong by
Wing Tai Cheung Printing Co. Ltd.

Foreword

Child Psychiatry is today becoming accepted as a branch of medicine in its own right. It is as yet, however, a young specialty whose characteristics are still being established. Early in its development child psychiatry adopted a multi-disciplinary approach at a time when nosology in general psychiatry was not soundly based. Moreover for several decades child psychiatrists have based their professional activities in widely differing fields demanding a wide range of experience and skills e.g. well-baby clinics, special schools, juvenile courts, psychotherapy clinics and so forth. It is hardly surprising, therefore, that the preparation of an introductory text on child psychiatry has for these reasons presented considerable difficulties.

It is one of the many admirable characteristics of the book, which Dr. Koupernik and Dr. Stone have written in co-operation, that hardly any traces are discernible of what could be called the 'identity confusion' of child psychiatry. Their clear focus on medical students may have helped to formulate succinctly the main methods and problems of the subject. The authors' wide experience and broad approach can be found on every page as well as in the composition of the book as a whole.

Although the orientation is clearly of a medical nature, I am confident that not only medical students, but also teachers, psychologists and social workers can profit greatly from this remarkably readable introduction to the basic principles of child psychiatry.

Utrecht, 1978   L. N. J. K.

Preface to the Second Edition

In the four years that have elapsed since the appearance of the first edition a vast amount of clinical study and research has been published. This has necessitated up-dating many references, as well as widening the scope of our suggestions for further reading, as requested by many reviewers. We have also heeded those who sought more information on the biological aspects of development, on the neuroses of childhood, and on psychopharmacology. The size and scope of the volume has not, however, been enlarged as we have tried to remain true to our original intention of providing an introduction to child and adolescent psychiatry, not a mini-textbook. A glossary of terms has been provided.

To our publishers for their friendly co-operation, and to Mrs. Hannah Kerr for her continued secretarial assistance we offer a special word of thanks.

Arduaine, 1978   F. H. S.
                    C. K.

Preface to the First Edition

This little book is intended primarily as an introduction to the psychiatry of childhood and adolescence for medical undergraduates. Throughout, we have tried to present principles rather than yet another quota of facts to be memorized. Psychiatry, we believe, can be effectively taught only by enlisting student participation in clinical tasks as well as in seminars. We hope that tutors will find our text a useful framework to clothe with clinical illustration, and a stimulus to discussion. We have assumed that the student has already acquired a basic clinical orientation, and has been introduced to general psychiatry and to paediatrics.

We should like to record our indebtedness to Miss Elizabeth Cameron, Mrs. Hannah Kerr and Madame Martine Léage, who have served our secretarial needs with patience and efficiency.

Glasgow/Paris 1974

F. H. S.
C. K.

Contents

Contents

1

Normal development

This book is intended as an introduction to the psychiatry of childhood and adolescence. As clinicians we are presented with a wide variety of problems of rate and sequence of development, of behaviour and attitudes, of deviations from health. In our capacity as family doctor, medical officer at baby or toddler clinic, school medical officer, paediatrician or child psychiatrist, we may be approached by one or both of the child's parents on their own initiative or at the prompting of others; the older child may request help spontaneously. Whatever the circumstances, we are always concerned with a problem occurring in a family group (or its substitute) within a community. As a basis for diagnosis we must be familiar with normative values, not only of the stages of development, but also of the mores of social class and cultural group, within which we observe the interplay of relationships and roles.

INFANCY

The most obvious external evidence of the rapid growth of the brain during the first year of life is the increase in head circumference from an average figure of 36 cm at birth to 46 cm at one year of age. This is of course a purely quantitative approach. Studies of brain tissue show that as growth proceeds, more and more nerve fibres become myelinated which means that they have become competent transmitters of nervous impulses. Some of the association fibres are already myelinated at birth. for example, those of part of the auditory system, which may explain the fact that the new-born already has an efficient though elementary auditory apparatus. At the present time much of our knowledge regarding the biological development of the brain is based upon mammalian studies. Among the endogenous factors identified so far is a specific nerve growth-factor within the nervous substance itself.

During the past thirty years there have been identified in the brain specialized sets of neurons each connected to a specific neurotransmitter. This is a chemical substance carrying information from one neuron to the next through the intervening space or synapse. These neuro-transmitters are formed from amino-acids present in food-stuffs, and go through various enzymatic transformations, the last of which gives rise to a precursor which is able to cross the blood-brain barrier. So far three neuro-transmitters have been identified:

1. *dopamine*, a catecholamine involved in the physiopathology of Parkinson's disease and probably playing a significant role in the pathogenesis of schizophrenia;

2. also a catecholamine, *nor-epinephrin*, concerned with sleep regulation, and probably playing an aetiological role in manic depressive illnesses in adults;

3. *serotonin*, an indolamine, which is probably also associated with sleep rhythm and possibly with manic-depressive illness in some patients.

These neuro-transmitters are neutralized by a complex set of enzymes, namely the endocellular monoamine-oxidases contained in the mitochondria.

Other important factors contributing to the growth of the central nervous system are those produced by the endocrine glands, the most important being the thyroid hormone, growth hormone, and gluco-corticoids. Recent work has shown that metals such as zinc may also be necessary for the orderly development of the brain.

At the present stage of our knowledge we have no absolute certainty about the importance of these processes in the development and activity of the human brain. One method of direct study of the infant's central nervous system which is available to us, however, is that of the electro-encephalogram. The classical work of Dreyfus-Brisac (1964) and others has shown that by the intrauterine age of eight months a difference in the pattern between wakefulness and sleep is already detectable. By three months of age there appear for the first time in the occipital region tracings which later develop into the classical alpha rhythm. Two months later this has become quite distinct.

It does not necessarily follow that all infant development and behaviour is biologically determined, but many writers have empha-sized that while allowing for individual variation, there is a predictable sequence of events in the early development of every child. (Gesell, 1940).

The newborn child is an extremely dependent creature and remains relatively so for longer than in any other species. Without a caring adult there would be survival neither for the infant nor for the species. Biologically then, mothering has to do with survival—a built-in drive to nurture and protect; in short to nurse. This is the start of the baby's first relationship, the basic experience of another being on which all later relationships will be built. And like all relationships it is reciprocal (mother-child; child-mother) as we may already observe in the feeding situation. The mother gently strokes the child's lips and cheek with the nipple of the breast or feeding bottle and this causes the infant to turn the head towards the stimulus and to begin sucking movements (*rooting reflex*). In breast feeding this sucking distends the nipple and induces the flow of milk which in turn by impinging on the back of the tongue stimulates the *swallowing reflex*. The mother's breast gradually empties till by humoral transmission the anterior pituitary secretes lactogenic hormone promoting the next cycle of milk production. As the feed proceeds hunger contractions cease, crying is overtaken by mouthing and sucking activities, the stomach fills and the bowels are emptied. With satiety comes sleep.

It may be seen, then, that this basic transaction between mother and infant is carried through by a sequence of reciprocal reflexes. They are functionally 'a couple' and not only at a physiological level. The mother 'talks' to the child in a private language of caressing sound, and as the sucking begins the infant's eyes fix intently on the mother's face, and his hand clutches her fingers or clothes. The child begins to know her sound, her feel, her smell; and she can distinguish his noises, and differentiate relaxation from tension. There is already the beginning of a 'feeling tone' in the existence of the newborn. Besides breathing, crying, sucking, swallowing, defaecating and urinating the child sees, hears, smells, and tastes, experiences skin sensations of temperature and is aware of changes of posture. Chilling, sudden postural changes, or pain may all produce crying, as does an empty stomach or peristalsis. Already two interwoven strands of development are discernible:

1. Reciprocal interaction between mother and child, laying the foundation for a system of communication of which language is the culmination. This contributes to the establishment of 'bonding'.
2. A recurrent cycle of phasic activity. Each peak of wakeful hunger is accompanied by crying, descends through an interphase of satiety, drowsiness, and murmuring to a trough of sleep or near-sleep till the next phase of arousal is heralded by further crying.

Although we can do no more than conjecture about the subjective experiences of infancy, the beginnings of self-awareness would appear to consist of alternating phases of pain and pleasure. Under ordinary natural conditions pleasurable experiences become associated with the mother's administrations and closeness; then later on she will be discerned as the one who may give or withhold. She is the first object of both love and hate.

By the second month babies respond to a smile with a smile, though without discriminating between people. There is some experimental evidence to suggest that somewhere between 6 and 8 months 'attachment' to the mother takes a significant step marking the point where mother is distinguished from other persons (Schaffer, 1971). From then on separation from her produces a sequence of distress, rage, apathy and grief characteristic of older children. Other members of the close family circle begin to be recognized before the end of the first year. Hearing reaches its full development at about 6 months at which time the child is able to turn the head towards a sound and thus to orientate in space. This is complemented visually by the ability, at 4 or 5 months, to follow a moving object with the eyes, and by *tactile-kinaesthetic* sense as the child begins at the same stage to grasp objects.

Direct observation of infants suggests that besides the eyes and the ears, the main sense organs are those of the skin (pain, temperature, touch), of the inner-ear (position and balance), and of the lips, mouth and tongue. The lips suck and touch, in this preceding the finger tips; the tongue tastes and feels, the gums bite and chew. These seem to be the earliest pathways of both pleasure and pain. There is now abundant evidence that for healthy emotional development infants require in addition to nourishment and protection frequent gentle confident handling by a familiar person.

Piaget, a Swiss logician and psychologist, has devised an original approach to the cognitive development of the child, that is the development of intellectual faculties. He identifies four stages as follows:

1. The first stage covers the first two years of life and is essentially *sensorimotor* and pre-lingual. Thinking and doing are not yet separate processes; the child's thinking is tied to his actions. This is followed by:

2. The *pre-operative* stage from 2–6 years during which the child begins to develop the power of internal representation. Language develops but to some extent remains egocentric and is not as yet an intellectual tool.

3. The third stage is termed that of *concrete operations* and lasts from 7–11 or 12 years. The child cannot yet generalize. This is the stage however when the child acquires the skills of reading, writing, and elementary arithmetic, allowing progress to the fourth stage.

4. This stage is that of *formal operations*, that is the adult form of logical thought. Piaget's main thesis is that children's thinking, possessing its own consistency, is different from that of adults. He stresses further that the sequences of these different stages is constant though individual children may vary in their rate of progress. (Beard, 1969).

EARLY CHILDHOOD

The transition from infant to toddler as the child enters the second year is most obviously characterized by major development in the skills of:
1. Locomotion.
2. Speech.

Sitting proceeds to crawling, and then to standing, walking and running. Along with the mastery of gravity, balance and co-ordination gradually improve. Continuing effort at mastery is observable as a form of 'play', and this in turn elicits from the mother and father a graduated repertoire of responses. At 3 to 4 months 'peek-a-boo' is a common expression of the beginning awareness that an object out of sight has not ceased to exist; as the child becomes familiar with its own body, mothers recite 'This Little Piggy'. The adult's tone of voice rises in crescendo in anticipation of pleasurable excitement, and, with the voice, facial expression, gesture, movement begin to be recognizable to the child as meaningful signals of communications before language itself evolves. Much of this 'play' of early childhood consists of a struggle for mastery of motor skills and involves running, jumping, hopping, skipping, climbing, throwing, catching, and so on.

The development of language, a uniquely human attribute, is dependent upon the ability to hear the speech of others, and to comprehend what is spoken as well as the ability to vocalize. Infant babbling changes imperceptibly to a production of disyllabic sounds ('ba-ba', 'da-da', 'ma-ma'). These merge into the first words, usually nouns or verbs which progress to two or three word phrases and then to short sentences. Tunes and jingles aid the process, and there is often an early liking for and imitation of rhythmical sound. By 6 months the infant begins to listen to his own vocalizations and to reproduce them. This is the so-called *circular reflex* (Baldwin, 1895). By constant repetition the child gradually associates a particular di-syllabic sound with the father or mother, and the first word is established. Ordinarily the baby's first recognizable word is not only a source of great joy to parents but held to carry a decisive developmental prognostic significance. In fact one child may use recognizable speech at 9 months, another at 18 months, yet this is no more than a reflection of the width of individual variation. If, however, by 2 years development is proceeding satisfactorily in all aspects, except speech, this is an indication of developmental imbalance and calls for investigation. Many children have difficulty in mastering the personal pronouns, and for a long time may refer to themselves in the third person.

There is no more controversial subject than the relation of language to thought and we shall not pursue it here, except to consider the so-called *negativism* of the toddler. Whether or not mastery of the negative precedes corresponding behaviour or vice versa, 2 to 3 years is often a time when parents are regularly confronted with the word 'No!'. Temper tantrums are common when a wish is frustrated and battles may be fought over feeding, sleeping, or toilet training. For example, young children like to handle the food they eat, and this, though usually harmless, may upset a fastidious mother; other parents are quickly made anxious if food intake drops, though in fact fluctuations in appetite are common. The 3 year-old may resist falling asleep and be very demanding of parental attention at bedtime; yet he may wake refreshed very early. Excretory functions have important psychological aspects. At an early stage there is an intense interest in the acts of urinating and defaecating, as well as in the products themselves. It is important to remember here that disgust and modesty are culturally determined attitudes which vary from one country and period to another. Babies and toddlers explore their own bodies and excreta just as thoroughly as they do their environment, and although this is quite normal, parents often need reassurance.

Many facets of toddler behaviour may be seen as the emergence from the helplessness of infancy to the first stages in mastery of locomotor and motor skills, of co-ordination of hand and eye, communication by speech, and sphincter control. The helping hand of the adult is progressively discarded; yet nearness of the parent is the only complete reassurance, and separation calls forth a response of intense protest followed by grief. The unknown arouses in the toddler both curiosity and anxiety so that there are frequent retreats from exploration to the safety of what is known. This may be achieved by having a familiar possession, a doll, a toy or piece of blanket or napkin from which the child may be for a time inseparable, especially when tired; or by the repetition of a familiar sequence of actions, so-called *rituals*. All sorts of situations and objects may provoke fear—silence, darkness, shadows, harmless insects, domestic pets, but especially being alone. These early childhood *phobias* may mark the onset of a developing neurosis, or be no more than transient phenomena (see chapter 6).

Co-operative activity with other children comes gradually preceded by a stage of co-existence, not always peaceful. Ruthless possessiveness precedes the notions of 'mine' and 'yours'; generosity and sharing are at first tentative and short-lived. Play still tends to be solitary with complete self-absorption in, for example, water, sand, and building-bricks. Group activity becomes a reality about 3 years. Now make-believe play begins to be prominent though for a time fantasy and reality tend to exist side by side, and many a youngster has created an imaginary friend or twin whose company is often very privately enjoyed over long stretches of time.

There is a kind of magical quality about the thoughts of most young children. For example, they tend to attribute human characteristics to inanimate objects which may be commended or scolded for being 'good' or 'naughty'. This is called *animistic thinking*. At this stage the notion frequently arises that what the child wishes is sufficient to cause it to happen—so-called *'thought omnipotence'*. Animistic thinking and thought omnipotence are encountered in some primitive societies, and may be observed in certain adult mental illnesses.

There is a curious paradox about early dependency, for in a sense the infant is a tyrant most of whose commands, conveyed by screaming, are obeyed with little delay. This is omnipotence of a sort in reality, not just in fantasy, and an omnipotence which must gradually be renounced if the child is to become a socially conforming being. It is this renunciation of power, experienced by repeated frustration of wishes, which is responsible for much of the rage and distress of the healthily developing toddler. As the frustrator is frequently the mother or father, each is often the object of aggressive impulses. Whether this proceeds with relative ease and speed, or with difficulty and delay is largely dependent on the parents' capacity to frustrate firmly and to contain the resultant distress with sympathetic reassurance. The child is frustrated also in one particular respect, namely in the wish for the exclusive possession of the parent of the opposite sex. Between the ages of about 2 and 5 years the intense attachment of a small girl for her father with rivalry for the mother, and of a small boy for his mother with rivalry for the father, form the ingredients of the basic 'family triangle'. Freud regarded this *oedipal phase* as a crucial one in the psychosexual development of both boys and girls. Whether the sexual component is accepted or not there is no doubt about the accuracy of the description or of the intensity of feeling involved. The attitude towards brothers and sisters, older or younger, but especially the immediately younger one so often the focus of *sibling rivalry* is usually compounded of jealousy (another rival for parental love) as well as affection. The resolution of these particular *conflicts* as with all the significant emotional milestones depends on the subtleties of parent-child interaction as well as the child's inherent strengths and deficits.

Gradually parental values become those of the child (*introjection*) and by the age of about seven years there is already established a self-critical faculty or conscience. In the process of its evolution the child is pulled between the strength of his wishes for gratification on the one hand and for parental love on the other. Here then we have a reasonable psychological explanation of the link between a child's experience of love, and development of character. Even more fundamental in the building of personality is the sense of personal identity, the awareness of self. At a very early stage the child begins to recognise gradually a demarcation-line between the 'self' and the 'not-self'. The neurologist postulates a 'body-image', the psychiatrist an 'ego'—closely related concepts, both of which involve the notion of a boundary-zone between self and non-self. *Identity* means the sense of being a unique individual, with a particular name, sex and role, and the formation of identity probably starts from birth and is not complete till late adolescence. The sense of being male or female is probably well established before the third year. Many factors appear to be involved, the attitudes and expectations of parents and others which include the conventions of clothes, length and style of hair, name, as well as the spontaneous imitation of the parent of the same sex; the discovery by the child of the bodily differences between the sexes. These, it would seem, are the external manifestations of deeper social and psychological influences, especially the parent-child interactions which determine the ultimate strength of personal identity. To what extent sexual identity is influenced also by biological factors remains controversial (Stoller, 1968). Parents of young children need therefore to provide both affection and limits, the basic ingredients of security, and most of them do so quite spontaneously, 'tuning in' to the successive developmental stages as well as to the special characteristics of the individual child.

LATER CHILDHOOD

Between the fourth and seventh year the child begins to emerge from the close protection of the immediate family. From then on each boy and girl begins to be able to stand alone, to tolerate with diminishing anxiety, increasing periods of separation from what is familiar and safe, to accept reassurance from other benevolent adults, and to enjoy shared activities with children of the same developmental stage. By the time the child starts formal schooling, usually at 5 to 6 years, behaviour has been steadily modified by a gradual fall in the level of motility accompanied by an increasing capacity for prolonged attention, as well as diminished distractibility. The child begins to be able to use a system of symbols, letters and digits, the tools of our civilization although, as Piaget has shown, logical reasoning has still to come. Participation in group-learning is now made possible by the ability to concentrate at least for short periods, some acceptance of discipline, more or less co-operative 'workplay', and quite basic to all the rest, the drive to learn and the capacity to relate with trust and affection to the teacher. For many fortunate children nursery and infant-school experience is enjoyable as well as educative, and can make a significant contribution to healthy personality development.

From now on it becomes increasingly difficult, and indeed misleading to make generalizations about development. Each boy and girl is now manifestly an individual not only in external characteristics such as colour of skin, hair, eyes, body build, contour of features—all determined by genetic endowment, but also in 'temperament' as revealed by the prevailing ryhthm of feeling, characteristic 'style' of gestures and mannerisms, in the evolution of which heredity and environment are closely interwoven. The child's position in the family, whether an only child, one of several, closely or widely separated in age from the others, whether an only son or an only daughter—all these circumstances carry potential significance.

Twins are particularly interesting. There are two varieties of twins. Some are dissimilar, dizygotic twins, that is siblings born simultaneously because of the fertilization of two ova by two spermatozoa. Nevertheless they usually establish a particularly close mutual relationship. Identical or monozygotic twins are the result of the duplication of a single ovum fertilized by a single sperm. While their genetic traits are alike from intrauterine life onwards there may be individual differences. For example at birth one twin may weigh more than the other. By law one is considered the elder, and it is common to observe that one of the twins has the more dominant personality. Moreover identical twins may live in a very private world and even develop a private language which cannot be readily understood by others. A number of studies have shown that the fate of monozygotic twins, even when reared apart, has much in common. In spite therefore of their being a biological entity, twins can not be regarded as completely identical persons.

In the older child play takes on a different quality becoming less personal and more conventional. Obvious is the element of rivalry as teams, organized or spontaneous, match each other in strength, skill and daring. Children often display much ingenuity in devising tests of individual superiority, and hierarchies evolve in competition for the approval of teacher or group leader. Make-believe and fantasy are expressed less in active play, more in listening to stories and watching television. The tales which survive, which captivate each generation in turn, the folk-tales and fairy stories give us clues to the themes of deepest emotional significance—the struggle between weak and strong, good and evil, the death of a loved one or hated one, heroism, loyalty, devotion, the mastery of fear. Drawings, and especially paintings, which at a slightly earlier age have usually been very colourful and personal, tend also to become conventionalized, often stilted. In tune with their respective identifications boys produce spacemen, cowboys, cars, boats, aeroplanes and space ships; girls, brides, houses, flowers. Only in dreams does the fantastic continue to hold sway. Meanwhile the acquisition of formal learning proceeds. Intellectual endowment is one determinant of the rate of progress but so also is emotional development, and early emotional deprivation can impair the capacity to learn. Group identifications are rapidly formed based on colour, social class and creed, and the prejudices of significant adults tend for a time to be faithfully mirrored in the attitudes of the children.

PUBERTY AND ADOLESCENCE

At the beginning of the second decade of life, puberty begins. The term puberty, literally the appearance of the pubic hair, refers to the bodily changes which characterize this metamorphosis. Puberty is an almost completely biological, endogenous phenomenon which occurs at different stages in the life-cycle of different species, mainly in the vertebrates and mammals. There is now a considerable body of evidence that what triggers the onset of puberty is the activity of the hypothalamus, but that external influences such as temperature, light, nutrition, and possibly psychological stimulation can hasten or retard this process. For example, in recent years girls have been reaching puberty earlier.

Hypothalamic activity stimulates the pituitary which in turn stimulates the so-called 'trigger glands', the thyroid, adrenals, and gonads. From then on events follow a different course in the two sexes.

In the male, under the influence of testicular testosterone and the adrenocortical androgens the testicles enlarge and spermatogenesis begins, the penis increases in size, and pubic hair appears. Axillary hair appears somewhat later, and last of all facial hair. The appearance of hair at these sites is due to a combination of a sufficient level of circulating male hormone and of hormone-receptors in the skin. In young adolescent males the beard sometimes does not appear until the late 'teens. In fact in some ethnic groups such as Asians and South American Indians there are probably no skin receptors, so that while just as virile as their white counterparts there is no growth of beard.

One other change should be mentioned in relation to puberty. The final growth spurt, which is probably due to a sudden increase of secreted androgens and which terminates with the final closure of the long bones, marks the termination of growth in height. Testosterone is responsible also for a characteristic increase in muscle mass. It is possible that this muscular development contributes to the characteristic aggressiveness of this stage of development in young males. Finally we should note the obvious voice change, the so-called 'breaking' of the voice typical of pubertal boys, which is often a source of discomfort and insecurity during the phase of transition.

Matters are more complicated in girls because instead of having one sex hormone they have three, namely oestrogen, progesterol and adrenal androgens. Sexual maturity is characterized by the onset of the menstrual cycle, and by a regular variation in the level of oestrogen and progesterol in the blood. The occurrence of menstruation at the end of the cycle means that the uterine mucosa has not received a fertilized egg, and desquamates.

At puberty the girl's body undergoes a characteristic transformation. Up till that time there are slight differences in the general shape of the female and male body. Puberty is marked firstly by the increase in the size of the nipples and then of the breasts. At the same time there is a widening of the pelvis and sometimes a tendency to weight-gain. Under the influence of the adrenal androgens the girl shows a typical growth-spurt, pubic hair appears with its characteristic female contour, and there is an increase in muscle mass though not to such a marked degree as in the male. There is likewise a modification of the girl's voice though to a lesser extent.

With the onset of puberty the boy or girl now enters the rather prolonged phase of transition towards adulthood, adolescence. Nowadays the 'teenager' tends to be the object of more adult preoccupation, anxiety, and generalization than at any other stage of development. Only in very recent years has a psychiatry of adolescence begun to emerge, and with it, the disentangling of those behaviour patterns which are transient developmental phenomena, from the signs of emotional ill-health. The physician confronted with the teenage patient has to take account of the self-imposed conformity, of clothes, hairstyle, and idiom of speech; and often to cope with provocativeness, defiance, or silent withdrawal. Yet this apparently near-homogeneous adolescent population is a collection of individuals, each apparently striving to conceal individuality. In describing some of the characteristic psychological features of this age-group we ourselves must guard against this current tendency to substitute stereotypes for real descriptions. Puberty marks not only the physical maturation of sexual functions, but also the accompanying emotional experiences. It is now well established that the onset of puberty has tended to appear earlier, 10 to 12 years being now a common age for the onset of menstruation, a little later for the first seminal emissions. These events and their associated secondary sexual characteristics produce diverse emotional reactions from anxiety, fear, even disgust at one extreme, to pleasurable excitement at the other, the latter often expressed as feigned casualness. The particular reaction is a reflection of total personality development (with its origins, as we have seen stretching back to the earliest years) as well as of the current relationships with other members of the family, and the parents in particular. Actual information about sex plays but a small part, except insofar as a complete failure of communication between parents and child, or gross distortions in the communications are reflections of disturbed relationships. But even in ordinary, reasonably well-adjusted families, many an adolescent suffers for a time from agonizing self-consciousness. The awareness of sexual attractiveness in others as well as in oneself may give rise at first to intense unease, concealment, or even temporary suppression. Phases of so-called 'adolescent asceticism' may alternate with compulsive masturbation usually accompanied by vivid sexual fantasy, and often with intense guilt feelings. The earliest emotional attachments are often to a boy or girl of the same sex, preceding the first tentative heterosexual love-affairs of the middle-teens. It is not at all uncommon nowadays in both sexes for sexual experience to begin in the early teens. Pregnancies in schoolgirls are increasing. Parents, teachers, and doctors are confronted by demands for contraceptive measures and even requests for termination of pregnancy, and find themselves in a dilemma where moral principles conflict with the realities of the situation. The problem may be further complicated by a tendency to malignant promiscuity, sometimes symptomatic of persistent drug-taking.

Alongside sexual development, goes the challenging of the standards, values and mores of adult society. Naturally this tends to be directed at the parents whose authority and prestige are under continuous verbal assault. Every firmly-held conviction or preference may come under attack especially in the spheres of religion and politics. Adult conformity is often designated as hypocrisy and adult prejudices are relentlessly exposed. No less disconcerting is the transience of the young person's particular convictions, and the swings of mood. Passivity, 'time-wasting', even profoundly depressive episodes alternate with phases of intensive activity, enthusiasm and high spirits. With disquieting suddeness very adult-like self-assurance may give way to child-like dependency. It is a time of particular strain in the relationship of daughters with their mothers, sons and their fathers, both with their teachers. It is hardly surprising that as maximal educational demands tend to be imposed at precisely this period of relative instability, poor scholastic performance is a common feature, even when intellectual endowment is adequate. Only too often this leads to scholastic relegation with long-term implications for the youngster's future prospects. The bewildered adult is often just as inconsistent, extreme permissiveness alternating with harsh coercion. It is not surprising, therefore, that whereas some adolescents tend to be solitary, the majority find complete acceptance with their own peer group. Paradoxically the group mores reveal a high degree of conformity, only the particulars varying from one generation to the next. While acknowledging the positive contribution that group membership often affords, and from which the adult gradually emerges with a sense of personal security and of purpose for the future, we must also recognize the widespread phenomenon of organized gang formation with aggressive and destructive activities. While areas of social, emotional and educational deprivation typically give rise to delinquency and sexual promiscuity so also may well-to-do middle-class populations. Much has been written of late about the material affluence of many youngsters and their consequent commercial exploitation, about the inadequacy of parental control and of religious influence, the menace of the overpermissive society, and the insidious effects of an adult world largely materialistic in outlook. Others lay the blame on the cynical indifference and hopelessness of a world divided against itself by race, colour, and creed, armed with sophisticated instruments of self-destruction, undermining any hopeful and constructive view of the future. Adolescent, and especially, young adult behaviour and attitude has to be seen not only in relation to the individual's stage of psycho-social development but as an interaction of the individual with a particular environment.

REFERENCES

Baldwin, J.M. (1895) *Mental Development in the Child and the Race: Methods and Processes.* 3rd edn. New York: Macmillan.
Beard, R.M. (1969) *An Outline of Piaget's Developmental Psychology.* London: Routledge and Kegan Paul.
Dreyfus-Brisac, C. (1964) The electro encephalogram of the premature and full-term infant. In *Neurological and Electro-encephalographic Correlative Studies in Infancy,* ed. Kellaway & Petersen. New York: Grune and Stratton.
Gesell, A. (1940) *The First Five Years of Life.* London: Methuen.
Schaffer, H.R. (1971) *The Growth of Sociability.* London: Penguin.
Stoller, R.J. (1968) *Sex and Gender. On the Development of Masculinity and Femininity.* London: Hogarth Press.

FURTHER READING

Carmichael, L. (1970) *Manual of Child Psychology*. New York: Wiley.
Erikson, E. (1950) *Childhood and Society*. New York: Norton.
Foss, B.M. (Ed.) (1965) *Determinants of Infant Behaviour*. London: Methuen.
Illingworth, R.S. (1975) *Development of the Infant and Young Child, Normal and Abnormal*, 6th edn. Edinburgh: Churchill Livingstone.
Isaacs, S. (1933) *Social Development in Young Children*. London: Routledge.
Koupernik, C. & Dailly, R. (1976) *Developpement Neuropsychique du Nourrisson*, 3rd edn. Paris: Presses Universitaires de France.
Masterson, J.F. (1967) *Psychiatric Dilemma of Adolescence*, London: Churchill.
Tanner, J.M. (1962) *Growth at Adolescence*. 2nd edn. Oxford: Blackwell.

2

The presenting problem

GENERAL CONSIDERATIONS

We are well aware that, situated as we are in Western Europe, what presents clinically is greatly influenced by cultural and economic factors. As we move into the latter part of the twentieth century, with ever quickening pace of scientific discovery it is well to recall that two-thirds of the world's population are continually faced with the problems of sheer survival. Where health programmes are confronted with widespread malnutrition, inadequate standards of physical care and community hygiene, it is understandable that child psychiatric provision seems an unthinkable luxury. On the other hand, where in the so-called developed countries malnutrition and infectious disease · recede and material standards rise, social, emotional, and educational problems of children and youth become more prominent. The factors responsible for this state of affairs, which, it seems, respect neither national nor geographical boundaries, are many and complex, and not fully understood. Wherever psychiatric facilities for adults, adolescents and children are provided they are rapidly confronted with demands beyond their resources. This is in fact one of the major unsolved problems confronting child psychiatric practice, demanding as it does a policy of clinical priorities, and realistic appraisal of treatment procedures.

Important also are emotional attitudes to psychiatric disorders. For many people the idea of mental illness in themselves or their offspring arouses feelings of fear and shame to a degree which is clearly irrational. Although attitudes are slowly becoming more enlightened many adults are still loath to seek professional help. Where children are concerned there commonly exist in parents the additional feelings of guilt and self-blame for the child's condition, feelings which may or may not be justified. It is not surprising, therefore, that the appraisal of psychiatric endeavour tends to extremes of disparagement or overvaluation. Psychiatric problems are discounted, and not only by laymen, as spurious, as not quite genuine, and therefore unworthy of serious attention or therapeutic effort. Childhood emotional disorders in particular tend to be dismissed as transient. It is true, as we shall see later, that the child does sometimes 'grow out' of the problem, but by no means always; and some grow out of one, and into another. If we are to help people to overcome their deep if illogical attitudes, especially when this interferes with the care of themselves or their children, we must remind ourselves that, contrary to frequent assertions, mental illness is often very different from physical illness, and that unusual, inexplicable behaviour can be very frightening. To have a child so afflicted may produce deep feelings of protest and despair. It may be seen therefore why the child psychiatrist must accept the often irrational attitudes of others as an inherent professional hazard demanding special qualities of tact and resilience.

Let us consider then in the context of a community with reasonably developed medical, social, and educational services how the psychiatric disorders of children and adolescents first come to light. Our headings represent the various sources of concern as follows:

1. Parents
2. Baby clinics
3. Nurseries and nursery schools
4. Family doctors
5. Teachers
6. Juvenile courts and probation services
7. Child-care agencies.

At the outset, to avoid misunderstanding, it must be emphasized that these are descriptive but not aetiological categories. Secondly, the groupings are by no means mutually exclusive, that is to say a particular child's symptom may be detected concurrently by several different persons, e.g. parent, teacher, doctor. Nor do we attempt to be comprehensive, but rather to give under each heading common examples.

1. Parents

There must be few ordinary, reasonable parents who do not at some time prior to the birth, experience a pang of anxiety about their child's normality. Every doctor and midwife knows how frequently the new mother immediately seeks just such reassurance. It is not surprising, therefore, that especially with a first-born, parents frequently express concern about the baby's rate of development. They may be worried that the milestones of speech, locomotion and so on are not up to standard, and it is probable that part of this concern is iatrogenic. Tables of averages still commonly in use can be very misleading in their failure to emphasize individual variation. Inexperience, lack of knowledge, or personal family circumstances may all contribute to anxiety about the child's intelligence. A particular and common worry is about the achievement of sphincter control of bladder and bowel, one manifestation of which is excessive zeal for early toilet-training.

Another source of widespread concern is the tendency of many children to display certain behavioural patterns such as head-rolling, rocking, thumb-sucking, nail-biting, masturbation—so-called *habit disorders*. These may be transient and of little account, or early signs of emotional disorder, a distinction which cannot be made on the basis of the symptom alone. When repressive measures are used by parents of very young children to counteract, for example, thumb-sucking or handling of genitals we have to consider whether the parent is displaying a sensitive or 'loaded' attitude, resulting in over-reaction. A little later the negativism of the toddler, which as we have seen is characteristic of this stage, may be misinterpreted as potentially antisocial behaviour. Fears of the dark, of being alone, of harmless objects and animals, common in the same age-group, and which usually respond to gentle reassurance, may be seen as evidence of a 'nervous child'. Parents tend to be less worried about the child who is consistently good, quiet and obedient though in fact this may be an early warning signal to the clinician. Of course, fathers and mothers vary enormously in their tolerance of their children, and this can be a very variable factor, depending not only on the particular stage of development of the child—there are marked preferences or ease with babies or toddlers, or girls, less often with adolescents or boys—but also on the parents' age, and health, physical and mental. Parental fatigue, worry, and illness may come to notice because of symptoms in the children. In some families there is a markedly low tolerance threshold for any hint of antisocial behaviour, in others for what is seen as scholastic failure, in still others for symptoms suggestive of physical illness.

What is presented as a childhood problem may prove to be a reflection of parental mental illness. The mother or father may display inappropriate or even bizarre behaviour, mood, or ideas, may be quite disproportionately concerned about some quite ordinary aspect of the child, may have profound feelings of guilt about the child's condition, may express fear of inflicting damage, or may be detached to an extreme degree. In such situations the child may or may not be psychiatrically ill as well, but is rarely entirely unaffected.

Sometimes, parents have no specific complaint regarding their child but come for advice about child-rearing practice—about discipline, rewards and punishments, feeding and sleeping regimes, sex education and so on. Such requests may be straightforward appeals for general guidance, or more usually for reassurance about the methods they have already adopted. There is, unfortunately, a growing tendency, especially perhaps in the USA and in Western Europe, for parents to turn to 'experts' in child-rearing rather than trusting their own judgement. The implications, that the skills of parentcraft are scientifically based, should, in our view, be resisted. The present reaction against the prevalent permissive attitude to discipline is not the outcome of new knowledge but a response to feelings of inadequacy.

2. The baby clinic (child welfare centre: well-baby clinic)

In the course of routine health inspection, developmental assessment and administration of inoculations, clinic personnel, doctor, nurse, or health-visitor, are frequently presented with situations which alert them to the possibilities of emotional or developmental problems. Disturbances in the mother-child relationship may be suggested by the persistent conviction that the baby is ill or abnormal, unmodified by repeated clinical examination and reassurance; by lack of pleasure in, or inappropriate ways of relating to the child. For an infant these constitute situations of stress, and may be responsible for reactions of apathy, of lack of interest in feeding, of vomiting or rumination, too much or too little sleep, excessive crying or none at all. 'Very good babies' sometimes prove to be abnormally unresponsive to and uninterested in their environment. All of these symptoms pose difficult problems of diagnosis for they may be indicative of a wide variety of physical diseases such as infection, brain-damage, metabolic or endocrine disorders. The fact that the mother is excessively anxious, disinterested or depressed does not exclude the existence of organic disease in the child.

3. Nursery and nursery school

As we have seen earlier the 'milestones' of development are not only of the motor and sensory varieties, but also of social and emotional dimensions. Nursery nurses and kindergarten teachers are quick to detect social or emotional deviation, for example failure to progress through the ordinary sequences of play. This may be due to dullness, apathy, self-absorption, or idiosyncratic play patterns; to extreme diffidence or even fears; to impaired concentration, or marked impulsiveness; to frequent tantrums or aggressiveness. Particularly alarming is the behaviour of the child who when some insistent wish is frustrated responds by breath-holding even to the point of syncope.

There may be dependent clinging to parent or nurse, or panic on separation from the adult. As with the infant one must be alert to organic deficiencies of the special senses, and of the balance and the neuromuscular systems, especially where there is clumsiness or over activity. This is particularly so also in relation to delayed or abnormal development of speech, in which hearing, comprehension, adequate stimulation, ability to vocalize, and emotional state may all be factors. Early psychological disturbance may be suggested by feeding disorders—food-fads, anorexia, gluttony or perverted appetite (*pica*); by reversal to wetting or soiling after a period of adequate control of sphincters, and by deliberate withholding of faeces.

4. The family doctor

The general practitioner may be consulted about any of the problems previously discussed, whether of development, behaviour or various forms of nervousness. In addition, however, he is frequently confronted with the child whose leading symptoms are somatic and for which he may suspect an emotional origin. In this category are disturbances of sleep, or appetite, recurrent headache, abdominal pain, or limb pain, restlessness, faints and tics. Secondly, he is frequently concerned about children with established diseases or conditions in whom there appear psychological complications. An obvious group are those children with visible congenital or acquired abnormalities of any kind which may cause self-consciousness, often more-so in the parents. The boy or girl with, for example, a limb deformity or an unsightly naevus may show little awareness until early adolescence when there is a greatly heightened need for social acceptance and conformity. This is also the stage when dull or retarded children begin to realize the significance of their disability, sometimes with marked depressive reactions. The problems of children with chronic physical illness and disability are dealt with in Chapter 6.

Less commonly the doctor is confronted with a child whose symptoms are frankly psychiatric in nature—worrying or frightening thoughts, ideas, or feelings apparently without rational foundation. There may be fears of strangers, animals, insects: of being poisoned, of dying, of danger to the life or health of members of the family. One must, however, be on the alert for the perceptive boy or girl who has a basis for such anxiety though unspoken, e.g. the parent who is a careless driver, a heavy smoker, or complains of headache or chest pain. Children may have obsessional, depressive, or occasionally paranoid tendencies. They may display calculated cruelty to a younger child or to an animal or pet. The paediatrician may observe that a young child admitted to hospital shows too little reaction, is 'too good' a patient, or in contrast a frantically obstreperous one. He will tend to look closely at psychosocial factors in children with repeated hospital admissions for accidental poisoning or injuries, whether suggestive of accident-proneness, or parental neglect or cruelty. He will be on the alert for the child in hospital who is not visited.

5. Teacher

Next to parents, teachers tend to have the best opportunities of knowing children well, of observing them at work, at play, in social situations, and of assessing their developmental progress. The infant school (5 to 8 years in UK) is well-recognized as a particularly valuable observation-setting for the detection of all manner of medical disabilities, of sight, hearing, comprehension, co-ordination, speech and so forth. Increasingly, however, teachers are learning to pay equal attention to manifestations of emotional disturbance in these early school years. Failure to learn may be due to intellectual dullness, or to impaired concentration as a result of anxiety. It may be a sign of apathy in a child from a deprived background or of linguistic as well as cultural confusion in the child of a migrant family. Occasionally there may be evidence of repeated, transient loss of consciousness in epilepsy, especially the less obvious forms of petit mal. Failure to conform (assuming that the disciplinary standards are appropriate to the age-group) may be due to a behaviour disorder originating in parental inadequacy and neglect, or to a hyperkinetic state connected with neurological immaturity—entirely different causation, but to a teacher the same problem, namely a child unable to keep still. 'Lack of response to discipline' may on closer inspection prove to be extreme negativism, aggressiveness or hyperactivity. A persistent state of anxiety may also be revealed in the classroom as extreme timidity, speech hesitancy, frequency of micturition, facial grimacing, or body tics. In the slightly older child playground behaviour may be particularly revealing—inability to mix or to sustain friendships, poor relationships with brothers or sisters, a tendency to dominate or even bully, extreme possessiveness and unwillingness to share, or impaired capacity for enjoyment. Frequent or prolonged absences from school may be due to a wide range of causes all demanding inquiry—parental collusion, chronic physical ill-health, irrational fears of leaving home ('school phobia'), of accepting the school setting or deliberate truancy.

6. Juvenile Courts and Probation Service

It is often fortuitous whether a child suffering from an emotional disorder is brought to notice by a physician, a teacher, or a policeman. Delinquency is a legal not a clinical term, and means behaviour in conflict with the law; aetiology and descriptive diagnosis can vary greatly. By no means all delinquent youngsters are psychiatrically abnormal at all, but reflect the mores of a sub-culture; it may be said with some justification that in such an environment it is the conformist who is deviant. It may be argued that basically healthy young people who become delinquent are victims of a 'sick society'. Probation officers and youth workers have come to recognize the antisocial child or adolescent who is an isolate, i.e. is living in a relatively non-delinquent area, and to be particularly alert in such instances for specific psychological factors in aetiology. Fire-setting (*arson*), not a rare symptom, also tends to be a lone rather than a group activity. Many of the juvenile offences are relatively trivial, and in some countries, for example Denmark and more recently Britain, are being dealt with in Family Courts or by Children's Panels rather than by the ordinary courts of law, the emphasis being on the assessment of the total family situation, and of remedial measures rather than punishment alone. There must be few readers who do not recall the occasional episode of truancy in their own schooldays; but persistent truanting is another matter and is often the starting point of a chain-reaction, leading to stealing, lying, car-thieving, and so on. Theft, house-breaking and vandalism are more often group than individual activities. Between gangs rivalries and feuds may lead to rowdiness and assault.

Drug-taking is a relatively recent phenomenon not only in adolescents, but also in school children. Adolescents may be charged with deviant sexual behaviour such as transvestism or exhibitionism; or with serious sexual offences, such as rape or homosexual assault. All such behaviour, whether harmful to others or not calls for psychiatric assessment. Children, especially girls may be victims of actual or attempted sexual assault. In such cases it is important that procedures such as gynaecological examinations, interrogation, or identification parades should not contribute to the psychological trauma. Sexual offences within families, whether assault, or incestuous relationships, call for expert family-psychiatric and social-work measures. So does parental violence or neglect. The child murderer is, fortunately, rare but inevitably creates tremendous problems of appropriate management.

7. Children without families
It is illogical that of all the children we have discussed those who are without families receive mention right at the end, which in many places is unfortunately a true reflection of their priority position for psychiatric help. Whether in children's villages, residential homes, or with foster-parents, as a result of abandonment, bereavement, parental cruelty or neglect, these children are inescapably a high-risk

group with regard to future psychiatric morbidity. Particularly vulnerable is the illegitimate child, especially the infant whose health or developmental status has prevented early adoption. Realistically with some 70,000 children 'in care' in Britain at the time of writing effective measures must be preventive. That is to say, children's psychiatrists and their teams must allocate time, not only for work with patients, but also as consultants to child-care personnel, and especially those involved in substitute parent care of infants and toddlers, and to the administrators of child-care programmes.

This, then, concludes our initial survey. It is evident that the service of the child psychiatrist may be called upon in diverse ways, and from many different sources. An effective child-psychiatric service must clearly keep under frequent review the question of priorities both as regards the needs of children, and the likely effectiveness of intervention.

FURTHER READING

Apley, J. & MacKeith, R. (1962) *The Child and his Symptoms*. Oxford: Blackwell.
Kanner, L. (1970) *Child Psychiatry*, 4th edn. Springfield, Ill.: Thomas.

3

Aetiological considerations

GENERAL CONSIDERATIONS

As with any other branch of medicine it is appropriate that we should follow the classical tradition and consider the why and how of the psychiatric disorders of childhood. There are two ways of doing this. The first, with the greater claim to a scientific basis relies on biological data or strong statistical evidence. Yet it would be naïve to believe that a single event or circumstance can always be regarded as *the* cause of a later effect. By this we do not suggest that psychiatric conditions do not have causes, but that in most instances several factors contribute to a particular situation. From aetiology we have moved to pathogenesis, from a narrow deterministic viewpoint to a multidimensional one which permits us to recreate the way things have happened and have become structured. Moreover, we prefer to think of 'conditions' rather than 'illnesses', which has precisely the false connotation of rigid entities. At the outset let us consider the relative claims of heredity and environment.

HEREDITY-ENVIRONMENT

That which is hereditary is by definition organic, determined by the nature of the genes. Thus we inherit for example our sex, colour of skin, eyes and hair, the whorl pattern of our fingertips, our blood group. Genetic endowment also determines the possible modes of reaction to situational experience. It may influence our liability to develop certain physical abnormalities and illnesses. In some such conditions, for example Huntington's chorea or phenylketonuria, there are associated disorders of mental or intellectual functioning. When, however, we come to consider, in the absence of clear-cut inherited syndromes, such features as intelligence, personality and behaviour, we find that genes alone do not provide a full explanation. While it is true that a child's intellectual development is limited by the kind of brain which is inherited, the extent to which this inborn potential is realized is determined to a significant degree by environmental factors. Much of the intellectual dullness in the population is the result of social and cultural impoverishment.

A recent example serves to remind us of the danger of oversimplification. When the double Y chromosome was discovered in association with both excessive height and aggressive behaviour in males, it was not long before there was talk of the 'psychopath chromosome'. This was subsequently shown to be untrue, and due to a case-selection bias, the result of the initial group of cases studied being in penal institutions. The familial tendency in major adult psychosis is now well-established on epidemiological grounds. The most conclusive evidence for hereditary transmission is seen in manic-depressive illness. In schizophrenia, while genetic loading is unquestionable, environmental factors are often significant, especially as regards prognosis (Wing, 1975).

A useful example to consider is that of the adopted child. Only a minority of such children develop personality and behavioural problems, but it is easy to see how readily these may be ascribed exclusively to hereditary factors, especially when something 'detrimental' is known or assumed about the natural parents. There is a persistent fallacy about an inherited tendency to promiscuity in illegitimate children. What is forgotten or overlooked is:

1. The crucial importance of the age at which the child was adopted, and the quality of emotional care prior to this.

2. Perinatal factors, especially if antenatal care was deficient, or the infant markedly underweight at birth—both common features associated with illegitimacy.

3. The quality of interpersonal relationships, expectations, and attitudes within the adopting family. (See also chapter 12.)

It is also important to note that many physical abnormalities which are present at birth or shortly thereafter are not inherited at all but are the result of pathogenic influences occurring during pregnancy or at birth itself; in short they are *congenital*. The central nervous system is very vulnerable, especially to oxygen lack, and particularly in dysmature infants. Factors to be noted in pregnancy are toxaemia, diabetes mellitus, abnormal placenta, air-pollution, irradiation and infection and misuse of drugs and alcohol. There is some evidence also that emotional stress at this time may produce permanent effect in the foetus, though the mechanism is unknown.

In considering the effects of environmental factors we shall frequently encounter the notion of *predisposition* in order to explain, for example, why a particular individual succumbs to a form of stress while others do not, why for example in an insecure family situation one child of several shows signs of emotional disorder. It is tempting to postulate, though hard to prove, a 'hereditary predisposition'. Of course the fact that a parent or sibling is similarly afflicted can be as readily cited in favour of the environmental viewpoint! There is increasing evidence that children are more susceptible to particular circumstances at particular stages of development: the infant to sensory deprivation, the toddler to prolonged separation from the mother to whom there is an affectionate bond, the young child to an ineffectual or absent father. When a patient is seen to be excessively 'vulnerable' to a stress factor, theoretically at least there are several ways in which this may be explained:

1. A hereditary predisposition.
2. Stress occurring at a critical period in the life-cycle.
3. 'Sensitization' by a similar stress situation at an earlier stage of development.

As we shall discover it is seldom that an emotional disorder of childhood can be confidently ascribed to a single cause. Often as the history of the disorder unfolds we encounter a cumulative spiral of innate and exogenous causation.

FACTORS IN CAUSATION

For descriptive convenience, we may consider these under the following headings:

1. Biological.
2. Psychological.
3. Social.

1. *Biological factors* are most clearly related to severe mental retardation, and to specific developmental disorders. They may be the result of genetic transmission, or the influence of noxious factors before, during, or after birth.

As the Isle of Wight Study has shown (Rutter *et al.*, 1970) children suffering from all forms of neurological impairment are more than usually vulnerable to emotional stress. What is not at all certain is why this is so. There may be a direct effect of the organic lesions by mechanisms not as yet understood. It may be that a significant associated factor is poor economic status, and that such families are more exposed to stressful life situations. Further, it is known that a handicapped child may readily become the target for rejection by one type of parent, or for overprotection by another, and that such 'relationship disorders' can of themselves lead to emotional disorders and personality problems. In the case of the 'battered child' syndrome, for example, it is noticeable not only how frequently one or both parents are immature, unstable people, but how often one only of their children is so treated, the one who is 'different'.

Very small babies (especially those under half their expected birth weight) are not only more liable to suffer brain-injury at birth, but are prone to behaviour disorders later on. In some instances this may be the direct result of organic dysfunction (for example in some cases of hyperkinesis); in others the fact of the child's prematurity may have been responsible for an exaggeratedly protective maternal attitude thereafter, a situation to which doctors and nurses may inadvertently contribute. Or again the prematurity itself may result from poor antenatal care and nutrition, or to exceptional stress during the pregnancy. Indeed the physical and emotional health of the expectant mother may significantly modify her emotional attitude towards the pregnancy itself, and her relationship with the child.

In discussing biological factors in aetiology we have inescapably become involved in social and psychological issues, a true reflection of the inter-relatedness of these various parameters of causation. It is therefore no more than bias to attribute all emotional disorders of children to parental attitudes, to hereditary predisposition, or to organic disease of the brain or other organs.

An assessment is seldom adequate for constructive intervention unless it takes into account heredity, previous life experiences, and current environmental factors. In short, aetiology tends to be multifactorial.

2. *Psychological factors.* We are concerned here with life events, with personal happenings or circumstances, how these are experienced, and the way the child reacts to them. Such factors are most relevant to the aetiology of preneurotic states, established neuroses, psychosomatic illnesses, and character disorders. As already mentioned they may be contributory elements in some psychotic illnesses.

When we come to examine the sort of causal happening or circumstances leading, say, to a neurotic syndrome, we attach greater weight to the continuing, day-to-day impact of a disturbed pattern of interpersonal relationships than to some overwhelming event of traumatic dimensions. It is true that the latter may occasionally occur, and especially if by misfortune several happenings overlap, i.e. if the child is subjected to cumulative stress, such as admission to hospital for elective surgery at a time when the mother gives birth to another child, or when there has been a major family crisis. Even in this type of circumstance we should have to examine carefully the total situation of *this* child in *this* family at *this* particular developmental stage. The neurosis of an adult caused by one particular traumatic episode in childhood which is subsequently repressed, and whose release in the course of short psychotherapy leads to immediate and lasting cure exists mainly, if not quite exclusively, in the imagination of novelists and film-writers. In reality, exploratory psychotherapy—which is indeed indicated primarily for the neuroses and related disorders—is a slow, laborious and largely undramatic procedure. This is understandable when we recognize that a crucial element in all such psychotherapies is the relationship established between patient and therapist, and the essence of treatment largely a working-through of the vicissitudes of this relationship.

We do not doubt that life experiences can be psychologically harmful, but we place the emphasis more on the impact of continuing relationship dissonances than on the fortuitous, 'traumatic episode'. If we consider two common and contrasting happenings of childhood (1) the birth of a young sibling, and (2) the death of a parent or grandparent, the subsequent prolonged disturbance which occurs in *a minority* of children so affected may hardly be attributed to the event itself but rather to the level of emotional security they have enjoyed during, after, and, especially, beforehand.

It has frequently been asserted that certain child-rearing practices influence emotional development significantly. An important role has been ascribed at various times to artificial feeding, early or late weaning, rigidly organized feeding schedules, early toilet training, the use of enemata and suppositories, swaddling and so on. We do not suggest that such matters are of no aetiological importance. It must be emphasized, however, (a) that the 'emotional climate' of the transaction is likely to be more important than the precise child-rearing practice, and (b) that children show marked inborn individual differences, so that what is appropriate for one may not be at all for another.

There seems little doubt that a child's emotional security is dependent on the quality of relationships within the family, and this includes the total family—parents, siblings, grandparents and others. Even in the modern western family, small in size and tending to insulation, the clinical study of relationships usually involves three generations. Basic is the relationship between the parents themselves. Where the marital situation is insecure, the family as a whole may move from one crisis to another, with recurrent disruption. Many parental factors contribute: incompatibility, poor personality resources, recurrent psychiatric disorder, disabling physical illness or handicap. Alcoholism, and drug-taking may complicate any of the above factors. Inevitably 'at risk' also is the one-parent family whether as a result of illegitimacy, divorce, desertion, or death.

Disturbances within the family can, however, be of a much more subtle and less obvious variety, and of quite damaging proportions, yet to the outside observer there appears to be little amiss. *Family psychopathology*, as it may be called, is by no means the prerogative of any particular social class. *Maternal overprotection* (Levy, 1943) for example, is a common middle-class as well as working-class phenomenon. This oversolicitousness may extend to all the children, in some instances as compensation for an 'unsatisfactory' husband, or may colour the mother's relationship with one only of several children, for reasons which originate in her own childhood and her relationship with her parents, with the circumstances of this particular child's conception, or with some attribute of the child himself. The overprotection may be a compensation for ambivalent feelings towards the child. Whatever the precise origins, the child tends to be exposed to inconsistent, even mutually contradictory signals, which lead to anxiety, over-conformity, and sometimes retreat. Development towards self-reliance is inevitably undermined.

By contrast a mother, while carrying out dutifully the child-caring tasks, may because of a deficiency in her own personality make-up do so in an unsupportive manner, lacking any depth of maternal feeling. One cause of such maternal inadequacy may be a history of emotional deprivation in her own childhood. Here then we have an example of a type of personality disorder which may be transmitted from one generation to another, but not via genetic pathways. This is one pattern of 'maternal deprivation'. Another is produced by 'discontinuous mothering', the infant or toddler who passes through a succession of caring persons, and achieves a stable relationship with none. Illegitimate and orphaned babies are particularly at risk in this respect; so also are those with chronic medical or surgical conditions requiring prolonged or repeated hospitalization. A particular hazard for very young children is that of *sensory deprivation*, that is where there is inadequate visual, auditory, tactile or kinaesthetic stimulation. This has particular relevance for medical and surgical techniques involving prolonged isolation or immobilization of children, as well as the responsibility of paediatric nurses to relate to the whole child.

Even where the basic mother-child relationship has been soundly forged, repeated or prolonged separations without really adequate substitute care not only produce characteristic syndromes of separation-anxiety, but sometimes lead to states of apathy and withdrawal. Such an infant may in many respects resemble an adult suffering from profound depression. A significant minority of babies and young children, emotionally deprived by separation suffer lasting distortions in personality development. The most severe after-effects are probably due to the cumulative effect of inadequate emotional care, separation, and sometimes physical cruelty.

Many of these different but related situations which are potentially pathogenic in the earliest years are preventible, but are still not given sufficient recognition by those responsible for the care of children in families, foster-homes, group homes, and hospitals.

The role of the father is also of crucial significance for children of both sexes. As we have seen in discussing normal development he represents for the son both an ideal and a rival; for the daughter he is the prototype of lover and husband. Fathers, like mothers, may as a result of their own disturbed or deprived childhoods have grown into immature, impulsive, self-orientated adults with little capacity to meet the needs of their children for affection and support. Children may instead be subjected arbitrarily to material indulgence as well as cruelty or neglect. They may be the witnesses to violence between the parents, and to adult sexual behaviour. They may be involved in incestuous relationships. By contrast there is the conscientious working father who in the guise of setting a selfless example is unconsciously pushing the child to satisfy his own unachieved ambitions. Indeed the father may be so busy being the good provider that his family experiences this as neglect. Difficulties may arise because a father competes with his wife for the children's affection by indulging them and undermining the mother's authority.

For many fathers a specially hazardous situation is the birth of a handicapped child. It is not uncommon to observe a father make quite unrealistic demands of a backward or lame son or daughter, and yet be in all other respects a responsible, affectionate husband and parent. Usually his behaviour is a defence against the pain of acknowledging the child's true state. In this respect many mothers seem to be more resilient.

There is considerable evidence that an ineffectual or absent father during a child's early school years is a common contributory factor to delinquency.

Though the aetiology of homosexuality is not well understood, the family constellation in which an assertive mother dominates a detached father whom she denigrates to her intensely loved son, seems specifically pathogenic. It seems likely that disturbed mother-son and father-daughter relationships are often at the root of sexual inversion.

In general one may say that when parental attitudes and actions are in response to the child's needs, that is, are child-orientated, there is unlikely to be much amiss in the relationship. When, however, the parents' personality is consistently self-orientated (*narcissistic*) the parent-child relationship is unlikely to be a healthy one.

Grandparents also play a significant role for the developing child. Whether this is a constructive one or not depends not only on their own personalities but also on their relationships with the parents. They may be supportive, acting as temporary substitute parents during periods of family stress, or fill a more long-standing need for the one-parent family. If, however, grandparents compete with parents, sometimes as a result of having been rather unsuccessful parents themselves, the child may be confused by the claims of divided loyalties.

3. *Social factors.* Where social and cultural deprivation exists children are psychologically at risk. Unemployment, poverty, poor housing, malnutrition can and do contribute to mental ill-health. Under such conditions the weaker families tend to disintegrate and children, especially in the earliest years are exposed to the dangers of *discontinuous mothering,* and of emotional neglect. Where the family survives as a unit this is usually a reflection of the strength of the mother's personality resources. In such circumstances an 'extended family' may act as a protective buffer while the nuclear family tends to be extremely vulnerable.

Severe or chronic illness in parents can have a profound influence on the emotional state of children. Quite young children often sense the anxiety, even if they do not fully understand, when a parent has had a coronary thrombosis, or operation for neoplasm; to the child parental depression may be experienced as lack of interest and affection. These three illnesses, coronary disease, neoplasm, and depression are the scourges of middle-life, when families tend still to be dependent, materially and emotionally. When there is bereavement, children need to mourn though in ways different from adults; especially they need support during periods of distress, anger and bafflement.

Psychiatric illness in a parent, or a grandparent living with the family, can disrupt the emotional harmony of the home in quite devastating ways. Irrational aggression is very frightening, not only to children; so also is excessive and inappropriate anxiety or irrational fear. A *folie à deux* situation may involve a parent and a child. Parental neurosis, while much less obvious, may nevertheless insidiously undermine the child's emotional development. That this does not invariably occur is partly due to the age and resilience of the child, partly to 'dilution' and support afforded by the healthy members of the family, and partly to the form and duration of the neurosis itself.

We must not overlook the importance of the child's physical health. Chronic illness of itself may contribute to emotional disorder (1) by its direct effect on the child, (2) by the reactions to an ill child of the parents and other members of the family, and (3) by the circumstances associated with medical investigation and treatment.

The breakdown of a marriage by divorce or separation will

inevitably affect the emotional equilibrium of all concerned. When, however, we come to consider in a particular situation what exactly constitutes trauma for the children we must take account of the quality of preceding relationships and events, the extent to which the father and mother compete for the allegiance of the children, and the role of relations and friends in affording support. Legal proceedings themselves may prove extremely disturbing, especially if the child becomes a pawn in the battle for custody.

In considering the psychological sequelae in the child who has been the victim of sexual assault, here again much depends on the child's emotional security beforehand, and how the situation is dealt with at home, and by the authorities.

The impact of migration, voluntary or enforced, depends on whether the family as a whole proves to be resilient and cohesive, able to withstand an inevitable phase of partial isolation, and to re-adjust to new language, customs, and surroundings.

REFERENCES

Levy, D. M. (1943) *Maternal Overprotection*. New York: Columbia Univ. Press.
Rutter, M., Graham P., & Yule W. (1970) A neuropsychiatric study in childhood. *Clinics in Developmental Medicine*, **35/36.**
Wing, J. K. (1975) Epidemiology of schizophrenia. In *Contemporary Psychiatry* ed: Silverstone & Barraclough: Br. J. of Psychiat., Special Publications, no. 9.
Robins, L. N. (1966) *Deviant Children Grown Up*. Baltimore: Williams and Wilkins.
Rutter, M. (1966) *Children of Sick Parents: An Environmental and Psychiatric Study*. Maudsley Monograph, 16. Oxford: Oxford Univ. Press.
Wolff, S. (1970) *Children Under Stress*. London: Allen House.

4

Assessment procedures

THE INITIAL CONSULTATION

From the previous account of the diverse ways in which an emotional disorder of childhood may present, it will be apparent that a flexible approach to investigation is essential. Depending on the particular circumstances the initial consultation may involve the child, the parents, the child along with the parents, and sometimes brothers and sisters also. There is no doubt at all that often this very first contact proves to be a crucial one. Nowadays when the public is more knowledgeable about psychological matters, parents still frequently betray reticence about revealing even to a professional adviser their anxieties about a child's emotional or intellectual development. This is partly a 'hangover' from the previous widely-held attitude that such problems were not respectable, that some stigma was involved; it is also quite often the result of irrational guilt. However sympathetic the interviewer, the father or mother may feel that they are under scrutiny as a parent, and that the outcome will be a verdict rather than a diagnosis. When parents feel like this it is not surprising that first appointments may be failed, that mistakes are made about the hour or even the day of the appointment, that the information given contains inconsistencies, that the attitudes are inappropriately defiant or, conversely, submissive. Sometimes there are clearly defined areas of 'blocking' so that no real information is forthcoming about a particular aspect of the history such as the pregnancy, feeding, or toilet training; the presence at the interview of a younger brother or sister may serve as a useful 'interference', and so on. It is only when one realizes that all these are protective manoeuvres, the expression of *psychological defences*, that one learns to observe them as useful data every bit as much as the actual spoken content. It is frequently objected that this type of interviewing technique is too expensive of time. In fact, half-an-hour will often suffice for a first interview provided the approach is a skilled one—an attentive listening attitude with frequent encouragements to continue; an attitude which conveys acceptance and interest, but which maintains professional 'distance'. Apparent irrelevancies are permitted (their significance is often grasped only later) with occasional gentle deflection. Brisk, incisive interviewing is to be avoided. There can be no hard and fast rules about whether this first meeting should be with the parents alone or along with the child. It is, however, not usually justifiable to begin a consultation by leaving a child in a waiting-room while interviewing parents, and occasionally the best practical move is to interview the child first. A common procedure in specialized clinics is for the child to be interviewed separately while the parents are seen by the social-worker.

Although a rounded picture of the family requires that the parents be seen, it is remarkable how effective a history may often be obtained from even a preschool child (except where there is extreme separation-anxiety). The child should of course be interviewed alone at some stage, and the psychiatric examination of the child will be considered in the next chapter.

It is not only possible, but often useful to conduct this first interview with the parents and the child jointly. Though it may be objected that it is inappropriate or even traumatic for the problems to be aired in the child's presence, in fact it is seldom that they have not previously been ventilated at home or elsewhere many times before. Often, however, they have been partially or wrongly interpreted by the child. A parent of reasonable sensitivity will avoid the expression of quite inappropriate material; in the rare cases where this threatens it may be necessary for the clinician to intervene. And a valuable clue has been obtained about the parental attitude. What then are the advantages of joint interviewing? Firstly, this allows the physician to define his role, as a helping person in relation to the family, the exclusive ally neither of parent nor of child. Secondly, it allows the reason for the consultation to be stated explicitly. This is often best introduced by asking what the child has been told, revealing frequently all sorts of evasions and distortions. Thirdly, direct observations can be made on how the members of the family interact with each other, as well as with the interviewer. With experience, a spectrum of norms is established in the constant setting of the consulting-room. For every family the situation is new and threatening, amounting to a stress experience. We are afforded, therefore, a first look at the family's coping technique, and thereby at their style of communication. Later it will be part of the assessment task to correlate what we have observed directly with what we have assembled in the history regarding family relationships. Though not essential, it is helpful to conduct this type of consultation along with a colleague, so that at a strategic stage, the child may be seen separately. Some psychiatrists prefer, however, to have an interview with one or both parents as a routine, prior to the child's first attendance. By so doing it is usually possible to obtain a more detailed and organized history, to assess more precisely the personalities of the parents, and the relationship between them. It is, moreover, a safeguard against the occasional untimely revelation in a family interview that, for example, the father or mother is not the biological parent, that the child is adopted and may not have been told previously, that a family member has a grave physical illness which is not mentioned at home, that a serious marital problem exists, or that a parent (or even both) is suffering from a disorder of personality or mental illness and may talk or behave irrationally.

The consulting-room should be furnished comfortably, informally, with some 'junior' tables and chairs for young children, and a range of play and occupational equipment readily available. If an adjoining or nearby play-room is available so much the better. Laborious note-taking is to be avoided though occasional 'jottings' are required by most. Confidentiality applies just as much to the child as to the adult.

Although it is obvious that a structured questionnaire type of interview-technique is incompatible with the approach being described, it is nevertheless essential to have an outline of the main areas of enquiry, along the following lines:

The presenting problem.

Medical history (of child, and rest of family).

Developmental history of child.

Schooling, social, and economic situation (preliminary).

Parents' own views on causation.

Previous professional contacts.

Expectations regarding help available.

Problems, subsidiary or additional to presenting one.

Marital situation.

Level of current stress.

Before considering these headings in more detail it must be explained that several contacts will be necessary, though occasionally a single interview can be used constructively. It is unusual to attempt to cover all these areas at the first interview whose main purpose is (1) to win the confidence of the family, (2) to assess rapidly whether a problem of sufficient severity exists to call for systematic investigation, (3) to determine whether the parents are likely to co-operate in a series of interviews if indicated, or whether their poor motivation or other material considerations such as travelling distance or expense makes preferable an alternative procedure such as hospital admission on a day or in-patient basis, and if specialist help is required (4) to explain to them, and usually to the child also, just how a child-psychiatric unit functions.

THE HISTORY

Having discussed the nature and duration of the problem one proceeds quite naturally to the medical history of illnesses, accidents, or operations paying particular attention to the child's emotional state during and after such events, reactions to separations by admission to hospital or elsewhere and how this was handled. This links up with the phases of the child's development which logically begins with the pregnancy and delivery, and the neonatal period. Where there has been delayed conception, a stressful pregnancy, a premature or otherwise complicated birth, early feeding troubles, a damaged or malformed child, then what comes first logically may be much too disturbing for early exploration. Here as elsewhere one proceeds from less to more 'threatening' material, allowing the parents to set their own pace. The child's development should be traced, not only the usual milestones of locomotion, speech and sphincter control, but also growth of independence, play interests and capacity, social contacts and group participation, attachment behaviour to parents and siblings. In short, one tries to cover the sequence of growth and development as outlined in the chapter on normal development. Eventually this developmental profile has to be placed in its context, namely what has been happening concurrently in the child's environment, and particularly in the life-history of the family.

In some instances a pattern will quickly emerge in which the phases of disturbed behaviour or developmental lag may be provisionally correlated with periods of family-stress, and often with disturbance or psychosomatic illnesses of other members. In contrast the child's developmental sequence may be recognizably deviant, in rate, quality, or both, with little reference to the overall family rhythm. Often cause and effect patterns will be quite obscure at this stage. It is here, of course, that the family doctor who has known the whole family over a period of time has a considerable advantage. He will already be familiar with the family's general social and financial status. At a first contact, by virtue of the physician's traditional role a direct enquiry may be made, for example, about the marital situation. This need be neither offensive nor insensitive provided it is handled in a cautious way, with the clear implication that an immediate 'confessional' reply is not expected.

In the discussion of aetiology it was emphasized that this is frequently multifactorial. It is certainly an oversimplification to consider all emotional disorders of childhood as merely reactive to parental psychopathology, disturbed family relationships, or sub-optimal child-rearing practices, though each or all of these may be contributory, and even primarily so, in particular cases. When a parent is recognized to be suffering from a psychiatric disorder the clinician must not assume that he has an automatic 'right of entry', or he may jeopardize any constructive action on the child's behalf. It may be necessary to proceed with the utmost finesse in the face of, for example, a father or mother with paranoid or other delusional features. Parents such as these may never consider seeking help on their own account, and the first consideration (apart from the welfare of the child and possibly other siblings) is to establish if at all possible a workable relationship within the inherent limitations imposed by their mental state. It does not necessarily follow that a parental neurosis or personality disorder is markedly pathogenic for the child though it will inevitably have some impact. These parental problems will be considered further in the chapter on treatment. When the problem has been referred to a child psychiatric department parents sometimes fear that, in taking the history, the psychiatrist is really investigating themselves by subterfuge. In a sense this is true enough, and is readily justified by the need to investigate all matters relevant to the child's condition. Yet there is an unspoken contract when a parent brings a child to a children's specialist, and it does not include examination and treatment of a parent in his or her own right by the psychiatrist, nor by the social-worker. This may be considered an academic splitting of hairs, especially today when there is increasing emphasis on 'family psychiatry'. We suggest, however, that when the focal point of a family disorder is located in parental psychopathology it is necessary carefully to assess how direct and explicit we can hope to be in initiating appropriate measures. The problems involved are both technical and ethical.

One will not necessarily meet both parents during these early interviews, even if this is presented as a condition of clinic attendance. Usually it is the mother alone who brings the child, often for simple practical reasons, sometimes with complex psychological motives. If the latter, it is better to sacrifice 'completeness' for a time, rather than force the issue. It is always advisable, however, when the father is not present to discover, if possible, whether he approves of the child's attendance, takes a neutral position, or has been kept in ignorance.

EXAMINATION OF THE CHILD

If a physical examination has not yet previously been carried out it is preferable to do so at this stage. This, however, is not always a straightforward matter. A very anxious child may be reduced to frozen immobility, or screaming protest at the first hint of an approach. To win the co-operation of a hyperactive child, especially at the toddler stage, calls for particular skill and practice, the examination often being completed only in several short periods, not necessarily on the same occasion. The same may be true when the child shows grossly deviant personality development, with markedly unusual behaviour patterns. Here the parents may be very helpful in anticipating what may be upsetting to that particular child, though apparently innocuous in itself. Usually one avoids the traditional white coat, or any display of apparatus and equipment. But one can hardly predict that a child is going to be terrified of, for example, spectacles, or black shoes, or broken toys, or the ring of a telephone, of being lifted, closing the eyes, lying supine, or of being undressed, let alone having the abdomen or throat examined. In the occasional circumstance where there is a suspicion that the behaviour reaction itself may be symptomatic of a physical illness such as encephalitis, poisoning or an intracranial lesion appropriate medical or surgical steps must of course be taken without delay. These special circumstances apart it may be assumed that nothing will be lost, and possibly much gained by proceeding slowly, and postponing further examination till the next interview, or the next again. Neurological examinations, in particular, demand the child's active participation. 'Difficult' behavioural reactions to the examination are neither as time-wasting nor as irrelevant as they may seem. The consultation is itself a relatively standardized situation, in which valuable observations may be made of the child's manner of responding to an unknown situation, and, as important, what role the parents spontaneously adopt. All this requires to be recorded along with the history and the findings of the systemic examination.

PSYCHIATRIC EXAMINATION
The psychiatric interview with the child is of central importance to the total assessment, and is dealt with separately in the next chapter. The important points to note here are that the child must be helped to feel at ease in this new surrounding, and realize that the physician is not a threatening person. With younger patients there is often an initial anxiety about being left by the parents or given injections. In clinical departments as well as individual interviews, group methods of observation are increasingly in use, especially for preschool children. One-way vision screens, while still much used for training purposes, tend to interfere with the spontaneity even of experienced staff.

Psychological examination
The contribution of the child psychologist is invaluable, especially when presented with a specific query. Routine administration of

intelligence or other psychological tests is to be deprecated. It is unwise to overvalue the significance of an isolated 'IQ' estimation. To be of maximal value the report of a psychological test interview should state among other observations:

1. How the child behaved in the test situation, and in particular the feel of the contact with the examiner. Hearing, comprehension, speech, attention-span must all be studied.

2. How interested the child was in succeeding in the tasks set, and whether there was response to encouragement and praise.

3. Where the child showed high competence and where low.

4. Unusual features, and discrepancies in the results.

5. A summary of the findings, initial impressions, and suggestions for further investigation.

Some circumstances calling for a clinical-psychological examination are:

1. Retarded psychomotor development.

2. Disorders of language development.

3. Educational failure.

4. Questions of personality development.

5. Vocational guidance.

There are now available a large variety of standardised tests, and the psychiatrist must be familiar with the main types of test procedure, what they set out to measure, and with what reliability.

Tests have been devised for babies (Gesell, Griffiths. etc.), for preschool children (Merrill-Palmer, modified Wechsler, etc.), and older children (Stanford-Binet, Terman-Merrill, Wechsler, etc.). In all these procedures the predictive value increases with the age when tested. Special tests have been devised for the blind, the deaf, and the paralysed but in all these the skill of the tester is of far greater importance than the procedure adopted. The Bender-Gestalt, Frostig, and Oseretsky tests are useful complements to neurological examination in the detection of minor degrees of inco-ordination, and of visuospatial disorders of perception.

Educational attainment tests are sometimes useful clinically as a measure of scholastic progress in particular subjects, viz. 'reading age', etc.

Projective tests aim to assist in the exploration of personality make-up, of the individual's modes of thought, attitudes to people, predominant feeling tone, and so on. The best known is the *Rorschach* or 'ink blot' test which has been standardised for older children and adolescents. Neither this nor any other projective test can be regarded as a substitute for clinical psychiatric diagnosis, and there is seldom justification for using such a procedure at all when clinical examination has proceeded satisfactorily. Where, however, a patient lacks all spontaneity, or resists any attempt at direct exploration, a projective test may provide useful clues. The Family Relations Test may prove helpful with young children, as may the Children's Apperception Test.

School report

For many children school is their first contact with the outside world and their adjustment to it a significant measure of adaptibility. The school setting is a natural laboratory and information from a childs' teacher can often make a valuable contribution to assessment particularly when there is regular communication between clinic and school, and when staffs have participated in joint discussions. Some clinicians like to have a free, descriptive account from the teacher supplemented by comments; others prefer to use a standardised questionnaire. The following aspects often prove to be particularly valuable:

1. General ability, educational progress, and whether there is good correlation between these.
2. Attendance record, and when there are frequent or prolonged absences, whether there is any acceptable explanation.
3. Unusual or difficult behaviour in the classroom or playground e.g. poor concentration, over-activity, social withdrawal, timidity, destructiveness (See Chapter 2).
4. Relevant information regarding brothers or sisters known to the school.
5. Previous contact with other agencies.

Prior consent for requesting a school report should be obtained from the parents, and information received treated as confidential.

Case-conference and reporting-back

The assessment procedure so far has involved a preliminary interview with one or preferably both parents, obtaining an outline of the problem and the overall history including the health record and previous contacts with other specialists or agencies from whom reports are requested where relevant; carrying out, or at least initiating the examination of the child by observation, physical examination, psychiatric interview, and psychological testing. The results of these various procedures now require to be collated by the psychiatrist usually by means of a case-conference with the clinical team. The sharing of different views leads to a provisional assessment of:

1. The type of psychiatric disorder, if any, from which the child is suffering.

2. The patterns of interpersonal relationships in the family.

3. The interdependence of (1) and (2), the extent to which modification may be possible.

4. The therapeutic measures or management procedures likely to be most appropriate.

In the majority of cases it should be possible at this stage to have a preliminary reporting-back interview with the parents in order to state the provisional findings. This is not only a mark of consideration, but allows for the release of intensely accumulating anxiety. This interview frequently becomes the occasion for the first uninhibited discharge of parental fear and guilt, and the establishment of a relationship of trust with the clinician. In retrospect it may often be seen to have served both, and yet the diagnostic process may still be incomplete. This is the occasion to decide on the need for further psychiatric intervention, and if so, to explain what procedures are indicated. If only the mother has been seen previously, this is the stage at which to request the father's presence. The interview may end by arranging a plan of treatment, or for a later discussion following further investigations. Before closing, however, the clinician is almost invariably plied with the very questions he has explicitly stated that he is not yet in a position to answer, viz. 'What is the outlook for the child's future?', 'Where have we gone wrong?', 'Is the condition hereditary?', and so on. The parents know that they can not expect immediate answers to all these questions. They are underlining the statement of their deepest worries, and ensuring that they have been heard.

FURTHER READING
Barker, P. (1976) *Basic Child Psychiatry*, 2nd edn. London: Staples Press.
Palmer, J. O. (1970) *The Psychological Assessment of Children*. New York: Wiley.

5

The examination of the child

Two special considerations make the examination of children distinct from that of adults. Firstly, the child is a member of the family group, and if the examination is to be meaningful, has to be seen in this context. It does not mean that our concern is exclusively with the father and mother (or parent substitutes), the child being relegated to a secondary role. On the contrary we lay great stress on the examination of the child, in his or her own right, but emphasize the integral importance of the family milieu within which growth and development proceed. Secondly, as an inevitable consequence, the motivation to seek help is usually that of the parents. The very young child has but a limited awareness of the purpose of the examination. The adolescent may without prompting be seeking help, or alternatively resisting frantically any such move. The middle age-group, the young school child, is often fully aware that the parents are engaged in a coercive strategy, and may accordingly present a daunting picture of passive resistance, which may extend beyond the diagnostic phase into therapy.

Undoubtedly some adults are intuitively more at ease with children than others, but on the whole child interviewing is a skill that has to be taught and learned like any other in the clinical field. Important ingredients are a genuine interest in children and their ways, the ability to communicate with them in a relaxed matter of fact manner even in the face of marked dependency, uninhibited rage, or calculated provocation. These extreme attitudes often prove to be reflections of the child's feelings towards the parents or other significant persons in his environment which have become displaced on to the interviewer (*transference*). Similarly, irrational factors can colour the clinician's attitude towards the child. For some reason, perhaps because he is a parent himself, because he has lost a child of his own, or identifies the patient with somebody else the doctor may, for no reason of which he is aware, experience positive or negative feelings towards the child (*counter-transference*). This is a common happening in human interpersonal relationships, but for a physician, and especially in the role of psychotherapist, self-awareness of feelings and attitudes is essential. Increased insight may be achieved by a personal analysis or by a form of individual or group supervision which takes account of this dimension as well as the acquisition of information and techniques (Balint, 1957).

Irrational attitudes of patient to doctor and vice versa may present in relation to physical examination. The student or young doctor is taught to follow history-taking by physical examination as a routine, but may be little aware of the feelings which accompany examining or being examined. There may be a vague recollection of his own unease during the early stages of clinical apprenticeship, but this is quickly overcome as professional objectivity is acquired. Many patients are noted to be mildly embarrassed, though much less so than a generation ago, some to be utterly confused, a very few, the exhibitionists, to revel in the experience.

Freud and many of his followers have emphasized the complicated attitudes to the physician which may ensue if his subsequent role is that of psychotherapist or psycho-analyst, and have recommended that the patient invariably be physically examined by a colleague. Today many regard this as an extreme view which holds good for only a minority of patients and situations.

Indeed, when a child, or even an adolescent is worried about some aspect of their physical appearance or development, especially sexual development, reassurance is often effectively and rapidly achieved by a complete physical examination. Occasionally a frightened or very shy youngster refuses to undress, and it usually is advisable to respect their wish until the matter can be discussed sympathetically later on.

THE YOUNG CHILD

Quite young children, even infants, may be referred for difficulties with feeding, sleeping, behaviour or parental anxieties about development. At this preverbal stage of development the examiner is dependent on (1) the history and (2) observable behaviour. Developmental diagnosis is closely interwoven with physical, especially neurological examination, augmented by standardized tests of psychomotor development. Ordinarily this is the province of the specialist paediatrician. Problems of relationship between parent and child, usually mother and baby, may have psychiatric implications, and may stem primarily from abnormality in the adult, the child, or both. It is necessary to observe how the mother describes her concerns, how reliable a witness she is, to evaluate her emotional state, and to observe how she behaves towards the infant, and what reciprocal communication takes place between them. The first hint that all is not going well is often obtained by the nurse or health-visitor during welfare-clinic attendances or home-visits.

With the 2 to 3-year-old it is likely that the examination will take place in the mother's presence. A few simple toys, building bricks, squeaking dolls, sand and water, may be helpful in making an initial assessment of intelligence, responsiveness, awareness of environment, ability to concentrate, dependence on and affection for the parents.

Sometimes an opinion is sought on the emotional state of a preschool child during a period of separation from home, for example while in hospital. Diagnostically this is fraught with difficulty, as the child's ordinary behaviour pattern, mood, and level of social competence may be quite atypical as a result of the reaction to the separation experience. With the aid of the parents' observations and that of an observant nurse it is often possible to assess how the child is reacting to the separation, but further assessment must usually be postponed till after return home.

THE YOUNG SCHOOL CHILD

As we have previously discussed it is often useful to begin the interview with the child and parents together. When the time is judged appropriate to continue with the patient alone, only an excessively timid youngster fears being left alone with the interviewer, at least for a short period.

Where the child has a readiness for verbal expression, conversation is the obvious ploy, the adult posing a few 'neutral' questions about the family, friends, school, other doctors previously attended and so on. A gentle comment about it being rather frightening in a strange place with a strange person may be acknowledged or contradicted, but usually serves to reassure. The unwilling talker may be offered appropriate play-materials. It is often useful to structure the interview to some extent and to provide the child with an opportunity to draw, paint, model, or to construct a scene in the sand-tray. Others prefer to tune-in to the child's preferences. By either method it is often revealing to observe the child partly in a free unstructured situation, as well as in a relatively structured one. A few standard activities such as drawing, painting a picture, making 'three wishes', and so forth can usefully be introduced.

It is not at all rare for the child in a first interview to be quite 'frozen', unable to speak, unwilling to play, on the verge of tears, or quite detached. Whether this is due to fear of strangers, of being abandoned by the parents, of being given an injection or admitted (usually re-admitted) to hospital, of being deeply depressed, or unable to make a relationship with anyone—will emerge only after further interviews. Usually the reassurance of having survived unscathed this initial ordeal ensures a more relaxed and useful interview at the next contact.

Every child at interview presents a complex and changing picture. Innumerable facets of behaviour and appearance may be noticed, some transient and irrelevant, others of major significance. The following headings are intended as guidelines:

Points to look for in the young child (preschool and infant school age)
Behaviour in the presence of parents, noting how child communicates with them, makes its wants known; how quickly and accurately these are perceived by the parents and how they respond.

Nutrition, level of care; appearance.

Child's attitude to interview room, and its contents.

Signs of fear, anxiety, panic, rage, pleasure—affect in general, and how it changes in the course of the interview.

Wish for and tolerance of reassurance and comforting by the adult, by speaking, being close, physical contact.

Interest in the place, in the play materials, and readiness to use them; preferences.

Acuity of hearing and vision; comprehension; skill in manipulation; verbal fluency, articulation, range of vocabulary; concentration and distractibility. Gait, posture, co-ordination, handedness.

Unusual or repetitive movements, postures, utterances.

Content of communications by conversation, painting or drawing, toy scenes, modelling—especially those produced spontaneously.

Account of dreams, day-dreams, wishes.

Expression of worries, fears, hopes, ambitions.

Talk about family, sibs, playmates, nursery group.

How child understands purpose of visit to doctor. What has been explained, and how much believed.

Acceptance of limits of time and behaviour.

Effect of fatigue.

Reunion with parents.

Child's reaction to first interview.

Response to offer of further interview (if made).

The older child (junior school age)
Everything mentioned above, modified for developmental level as appropriate.

Friends, leisure activities, youth clubs.

Range of interests and knowledge.

Rough assessment of educational level (comic papers, picture and story books useful).

Attitude to schoolteacher.

What sort of help, if any, is expected from clinic attendance.

The most dreaded outcome of interview.

Degree of trust in the adult, willingness to confide, understanding of meaning of confidentiality.

The adolescent

Pubertal status.

Affective state; anxiety, depression, hypomania.

Evidence of thought disorder.

Own version of problem.

Attitude to help being sought.

Emotional ties with family.

Friends, love-life, leisure interests.

Educational level.

Plans for future.

Every interview with a child (as indeed with an adult) is a unique experience, and the interviewer should emerge knowing (at least to some extent) a person, and not merely possessing a collection of clinical data. Extensive experience is required of the range of individual variation at successive maturational levels before diagnostic expertise can be acquired. Sometimes a child's behaviour is so disorganized as to make methodical work impossible, but this in itself is diagnostically useful. Equally frustrating is the child who is so rigidly controlled in behaviour and responses that it is difficult to gain any real view of the individual concealed behind these *defences*.

Children are not nearly as able to conceal themselves in this and similar ways in the years up to about 7 or 8 so that the content of interviews with the younger age-groups tend to be richer, less inhibited, and more revealing. From about 8 to 12 years, control and formality are often in evidence so that the interviewer who seeks to look 'below the surface' has to rely on the spontaneous production of stories, poems, paintings, and sometimes dreams. None of these may be forthcoming. Even the responses to projective tests may be so formal as to be quite unrevealing—except for the fact that defences are being strongly maintained. Moreover, the doctor, and even more so the psychiatrist, is seen by the school child as a representative of adult society, as an authority figure to be dealt with accordingly. In what precise way depends upon the child's previous experience with figures in authority, foremost the parents and especially the father, as well as the family's attitude to society and its rules. This is particularly relevant in the case of conduct disorders and learning difficulties which together make up a major proportion of the problems affecting this age range.

Around puberty there is often a relative loosening of defences so that access to the inner thoughts and feelings again becomes easier, though now we have often to deal with the extreme self-consciousness, embarrassment, emotionality, and indeed vulnerability of the young adolescent.

Any boy or girl may be concealing behind a 'front' of sullenness, unconcern, or defiance intense feelings of guilt and even depression, and yet be quite unable to communicate these to the parents. This may be due to inability or unwillingness of the parent to understand and support, or it may be due essentially to the extreme constraint which is characteristic of many young people. It may be easier to talk to a concerned stranger in a consulting-room, one who is prepared to listen as the story unfolds slowly, often hesitantly over a series of talks. The relationship of trust is the first priority. Sometimes this process of unburdening starts quite early in the contact, so that diagnosis merges with therapy. It is both unrealistic and inappropriate to expect the psychiatric process inevitably to follow the medical one of diagnosis preceding treatment. Both often proceed in an interwoven pattern.

The adolescent has to be approached with tact, even delicacy. His situation in the modern world is a peculiar one. His intelligence, emotions, sexual drives are more or less adult, and yet he remains dependent, inexperienced, and prone to panic or aggressive reactions, just like a younger child. At interview he must be assured of confidentiality, and even if he has not attained legal maturity has the right to benefit from professional secrecy. The safety of the patient and of others must of course be taken into account.

Some adolescents can verbalize their worries, others have to be helped. Some behave in a hostile, negativistic, even aggressive manner, and may not hesitate to insult their physician. This attitude towards adults may be a reflection of their emotional problem, may be a symptom of mental illness, and occasionally may happen under the provocation of an insensitive or unnecessary interview.

Any suggestion of disorientation in time or space should lead to a careful search for a neurological or toxic state. This apart, there is seldom a pressing need to reach a very precise 'diagnosis'. What is important is to evaluate the situation in order to take appropriate steps. Usually it is constructive to involve the teenage boy or girl in this decision in order to establish an alliance. This can usually be done without undermining parental authority.

REFERENCE

Balint, M. (1957) *The Doctor, his Patient, and the Illness*. London: Pitman.

FURTHER READING

Stone, F. H. (1976) *Psychiatry and the Paediatrician*. London: Butterworths.

6

Healthy and neurotic responses

Numerous attempts have been made to devise a classification of childhood psychiatric disorders, none of them very satisfactory. This is true also of psychiatric disorders in general. To some extent the subject has a certain intrinsic lack of precision. Clinical features which are reasonably well defined such as anxiety, depression or immaturity, elude quantification, and a subject which defies measurement is by many denied the status of a science, albeit a clinical science. Perhaps some day we shall discover precise techniques of measurement, replace woolly terms like 'love' and 'hate' with biochemical or biophysical equivalents, and acquire scientific 'respectability'. It is also possible that the more we learn about human thought, emotions, and behaviour the less appropriate will be the traditional methods of physical sciences. For the present, the physician who specializes in psychiatry is most effective as well as realistic, who readily tolerates the uncertain and the imprecise.

One of the greatest difficulties, irrespective of the age-group we study, is that of defining normality. Every branch of medicine, and especially psychological medicine, recognizes the importance of individual variation. If we consider for example the range of intelligence in the community, it is obviously a quite arbitrary matter where we delineate the boundary between 'dull normal' intelligence and 'borderline mental retardation'. How much more complex it becomes when we try to devise grades of 'personality strength'! When we consider children and adolescents our difficulties are increased. Besides the individual variation from child to child, we have to take into account the stage and rate of development. Unless we have very reliable historical, maturational data, this demands observation over a period of time.

The following criteria of emotional health are suggested as guidelines in the clinical psychiatric examination of a child or adolescent:
1. Development is moving forward; it is neither stationary nor going backwards.
2. Within the particular cultural and social setting achievements and

interests are appropriate to age and sex.

3. There is recognizable capacity for imagination, and phantasy, as well as ability to distinguish this from reality.

4. There is evidence of the ability to give and receive love.

5. There is ability to tolerate stress and frustration, and a flexible range of coping mechanisms.

In attempting to make a prognosis these attributes taken together often provide a valuable adjunct to symptomatology and diagnostic category.

Classification

The student may find useful the following classification of childhood psychiatric disorders which is a slightly simplified version of that prepared by the Group for the Advancement of Psychiatry (1968).

    I Aspects of normal development (healthy responses)
   II Stress reactions (reactive disorders)
  III Neuroses
  IV Psychosomatic disorders
   V Developmental problems
  VI Personality disorders
 VII Psychoses
VIII Brain syndromes
  IX Mental handicap

ASPECTS OF NORMAL DEVELOPMENT (HEALTHY RESPONSES)

Many of the 'emotional problems' of childhood and adolescence are in fact no more than the ordinary vicissitudes of development. In the opening chapter we have highlighted many quite healthy and ordinary developmental features which give rise to concern either because the parent has erroneous ideas of normality, or for some reason has a very low tolerance threshold. As regards parental attitudes, in fifty years the pendulum has swung from the restrictive to the permissive extreme, although the characteristics of childhood development have remained the same. By and large babies tend to be imperious, toddlers demanding, 10-year-olds guarded, and adolescents labile, irrespective of the currently fashionable attitude towards behaviour. Many inexperienced parents are quite unaware of the great variation between healthy babies in, for example, their sleep requirements. Some sleep a great deal, others very little; with some their waking/sleeping rhythm is decidedly inconvenient without in fact being abnormal. There are also marked individual differences in activity level which call for appropriate techniques of nursing and feeding. Most babies explore their bodies diligently—their hands, their feet, their orifices, their genitals, and occasionally parents are unnecessarily alarmed lest this should presage sexual abnormality. Thumb-sucking, rocking, masturbation are all commonly seen as transient features in perfectly normal babies and toddlers. When such a habit becomes prolonged it serves as a danger signal and calls for an examination of the child's emotional development. Persistent habits of self-gratification (*auto-erotism*) may be symptomatic of insecurity, unhappiness, or a sign of an emotional disorder. Wide variations in appetite are also common; so are temporary food-fads, with dislike of particular consistencies, flavours, or even colours; spontaneous vegetarianism is quite common, sometimes an altruistic reaction to animal slaughter, sometimes a reflection of high anxiety about aggression in general. The *negativism* of toddlers is so common as to be regarded as typical of this phase of development, at least in our culture. It is the inevitable response to the curbing of infantile demands. As we have discussed earlier, limits are as essential to the developing child as is security and affection. Overpermissiveness leads to anxiety and persistent *testing out*, a character profile recognized by the layman as 'a spoilt child'.

There is also much individual variation in the acquisition of sphincter control. Many are 'out of nappies' during the day by 18 months to 2 years; most are dry at night by 2 to 3 years, and bowel control is usually confidently achieved about the same stage. Occasional 'accidents' are, however, common for a time. It is doubtful if voluntary sphincter control is ever physiologically possible before 12 months.

Dolls and teddy-bears, and sometimes playthings can be a source of comfort to a child, a particular one sometimes being chosen for this function till it becomes an indispensable accompaniment. An interesting variation is the piece of material, usually fringed and with a distinctive texture to which many youngsters become attached, especially at times of discomfort or anxiety, and to which they often give a pet name. This 'transitional object' (Winnicott, 1958) tends to be given up after a few months, but is occasionally retained for years.

Another common phenomenon in the preschool or early school-age child is the 'imaginary companion' with whom the child lives throughout the day, sharing experiences in animated conversation with a consistency which can be delightful but sometimes alarming. This is often an example of normal *phantasy activity* of early childhood, though in an adult it might be regarded as evidence of a psychotic illness. Whereas the capacity for *reality testing* serves as a basic criterion of sanity in the adult, with young children we have to note that there is an undifferentiated stage in the second, third and fourth years, where reality and phantasy can and often do exist side by side.

Great concern is occasionally aroused when, around the age from 3 to 6 years small boys show marked preference for feminine activities, toys, or even clothes. This is usually evidence of passing imitation of and identification with the mother, which gives way in a short time to masculine traits. Likewise but somewhat later girls are often for a time markedly tomboyish and unfeminine, but outgrow this completely. When such inverted traits persist for a year or more they should be given attention, for it is probable that the earliest manifestations of transvestism appear before puberty.

All these are examples of the wide variation in the developmental features of ordinary children which often, however, are brought to doctors as matters of concern. Another source of difficulty is when the parents' perception or judgment is biased as a result of emotional disorder. This we shall return to in discussing family psychiatry.

STRESS REACTIONS (REACTIVE DISORDERS)

Here the child's behaviour is a transient reaction to current environmental stress, the relief of which results in the disappearance of the symptom. Stress means different things at different stages. Babies become upset as a result of tense or insecure handling, and respond with disturbances in the pattern of feeding, sleeping or crying. From about 6 months to 3 years there is marked sensitivity to being alone, especially with strangers, and prolonged separation from parents produces a characteristic sequence of protest, despair, and detachment. (Spitz, 1946; Bowlby, 1972) From this stage on, the move to a new home, the birth of a sibling, the death of a member of the family group can all produce temporary anxiety and insecurity, with a wide range of associated symptoms such as increased dependency, loss of interest in food, sleep disturbance, and loss of sphincter control (*emotional regression*). Provided these infantile traits are handled sympathetically there is usually a rapid and complete recovery. In the older child stress may be due to unrealistic expectations for achievement from ambitious parents or teachers, even 'blindness' to the existence of a handicap. Stress may result from domestic violence, or the presence of more than one mother figure, in competition or conflict. The onset of puberty may contribute a major stress situation for one child, a minimal one for another, depending upon (a) how successfully emotional development has proceeded till then and (b) the quality of support and understanding from the parents. Stress reactions in some individuals take the form of mild, transient psychosomatic illnesses.

Everyone has characteristic and very personal ways of coping with stress. These coping or *defence mechanisms* can be observed even in very young children. They form an important component of play, in which the child gradually comes to terms with a strange or frightening situation or happening. Typical examples are 'playing at school', or 'going to the dentist' in which the child acts the part of the feared adult (*identification with the aggressor*). Bed-time *rituals* are another common device by which a timid child creates a reassuring familiarity through repetition of actions or sayings. Other coping mechanisms commonly seen are temporary emotional withdrawal, or episodic hyperactivity and elation (*hypomania*). It is a sign of a resilient personality that a reasonable degree of stress can be tolerated without invariable recourse to a restricted mode of reaction. This is what was meant previously by 'a flexible range of coping mechanisms'.

The degree of reaction to a stressful situation may be increased by a previous similar situation, the individual having become 'sensitised'. Such 'sensitisations' may become built into the person's character structure, resulting in a tendency to over-react towards, for example, authority figures, rivalry situations, personal slights, or loss of friendship.

THE NEUROSES

The neuroses (psychoneuroses) are among the commonest forms of psychiatric disorder occurring in adults. In contrast to the psychoses, the major mental illnesses, the neuroses are often mild, and are not characterised by disorder of thought, or loss of contact with reality. That is not to say, however, that the thoughts, attitudes, ideas of the neurotic patient are always rational. Moreover, a neurotic illness may sometimes be both prolonged and disabling, in contrast to some brief psychotic episodes. In adults, the particular form of neurotic illness can usually be fairly easily identified by the predominant symptomatology as one of the following:

Anxiety state
Phobia
Reactive depression
Hysteria
Obsessive-compulsive state

In children, however, especially before puberty, mixed types are usual, precursors of the 'crystallised' adult forms. For this reason, some clinicians prefer the term 'emotional disorders'. There is no hard and fast dividing line between these and the foregoing 'stress reactions', though in retrospect the neuroses are seen to be more prolonged and to be little influenced by 'environmental manipulation'.

Anxiety States are characterized by subjective feelings of distress, with somatic manifestations of sweating, tachycardia, hyperpnoea and sometimes abdominal colic, occurring without any identifiable cause. Such attacks may frequently occur when walking in the street, and untreated may result in the patient becoming housebound. (agoraphobia) They may take the form of panic attacks, and may occur as early as the third or fourth year of life, when the child seeks out and clings to the nearest available parent or familiar adult. Like the adult the afflicted child can give no explanation. In middle childhood the anxiety may be sufficiently severe to prevent the child leaving home in the morning to attend school.

School refusal though occasionally symptomatic of a bereavement reaction or very rarely an early manifestation of schizophrenia, is usually evidence of a childhood anxiety neurosis. Irrational fears, for example about the welfare of the parents, are common though not always readily acknowledged. The anxiety is more likely to be about leaving home i.e. separation from parent, than anything in school itself. A pre-requisite for the successful understanding and management of the problem is to view the child patient in the context of the family. Invariably one discovers unresolved tensions in family interactions, though often well disguised. A treatment plan must involve parents as well as child. Essential ingredients are the building up of trust with the family, temporary emotional support, and insight-giving techniques by means of case-work and psychotherapy. Out-patient management is to be preferred; in resistant cases a programme of day-attendance to child-guidance clinic or day-hospital may be indicated. A period of in-patient care may be required as a planned phase of treatment. Rarely it is necessary to recommend admission to a specially staffed residential-school.

A phobia is a circumscribed form of neurotic anxiety, an intense fear without rational basis of a particular object or situation. Minor phobias are so common in pre-school children, generally resolving spontaneously, that it is doubtful whether they should be classed as neuroses at all. Common examples are intense fears of shadows, of feathers, of insects or of domestic pets. These phobias are not necessarily the result of actual experiences e.g. of being stung or bitten, but may be the outcome of intensely felt emotions such as anger, jealousy and fear, usually in relation to parents or siblings, intensified and often subsequently distorted in the child's phantasy.

When deeply felt but opposing wishes are present at the one time without rapid resolution the resultant *conflict* is experienced as an extremely unpleasant feeling. From this anxiety the individual seeks to escape by some psychological manoeuvre involving the use of defence mechanisms. If, for example, a child imagines that a loved parent is rejecting and angry, perhaps in response to the child's badness, the parental anger may be ascribed instead to some harmless domestic pet. None of this, however, is necessarily apparent to the onlooker who observed only that the child has suddenly and inexplicably developed an intense fear of, for example, a previously loved puppy ('dog phobia'). Others prefer to view these symptoms as evidence of faulty learning or adaptation responses, and accordingly favour an operant conditioning approach to treatment. These differing viewpoints are probably not as incompatible as are sometimes thought.

Depression often occurs in association with anxiety. Neurotic or *reactive depression* is so termed in distinction to *endogenous depression* though they are more likely to represent extremes of a continuum than truly separate entities. Whereas manic-depressive psychosis is extremely rare before puberty, reactive depression occurs quite commonly in childhood. (See chapter 9) The symptoms are similar to those in the adult, anorexia, insomnia, apathy, and sometimes hypochondriasis, but the slowing down of reaction-time, of speech and bodily movement (*psycho-motor retardation*) tends to be much less obvious. Children may be as affected as adults by the loss of a loved person or even of a favourite pet, and in the same way as the grown-up need additional support during the period of mourning. Anti-depressant drugs are no substitute for these special measures, though they may occasionally be indicated for additional symptomatic relief. (See chapter 11) There is now a good deal of evidence that for many children parental separation or divorce has more long-term effects than the death of a parent.

Hysteria in adults occurs much less frequently in Western Europe than in former years. Indeed it is somewhat suspect as a diagnostic category, not only because of the possibility of unidentified organic disease, but also because there may be an alternative, more sound, psychiatric formulation. We believe that hysteria is a real entity, which may take the form of stupor, of fits, of prolonged periods of 'dissociation' (fugues), or of loss of bodily function such as paralysis, aphonia, deafness, blindness, or localised anaesthesia. All of these hysterical manifestations can occur in children but none are common. The psychodynamic explanation of these symptoms is that a repressed unresolved conflict is 'converted' into a bodily symptom, thus the term *conversion hysteria*. Significance is attached to:

1. The time of onset—any significant happening which has acted as a 'trigger'.

2. The symbolic meaning of the symptom e.g. having overheard something which is distressingly unwelcome, loss of hearing follows (hysterical deafness); being unable to choose between divorced parents a teenage girl loses the ability to walk (hysterical paralysis).

3. The 'chosen' symptom may have been a characteristic of someone with whom the patient has or had an intense but ambivalent relationship (hysterical identification).

Obsessive-compulsive states are the forms of neurosis most resistant to treatment. Recently it has been claimed that behaviour therapy produces better results than other forms of psychotherapy or drug treatment, but this is not yet fully established. A typical adult compulsive symptom is repetitive hand-washing, which however lessens the conviction of being unclean only very temporarily. This is occasionally encountered in children, though seldom under five or six years of age. Obsessional thoughts, that is constant rumination on one particular, usually guilt-laden theme, may also though rarely occur in children. Anxious children sometimes display obsessionally tidy and meticulous behaviour, for example with regard to the appearance of clothing or preparation of written school-work. This may be described by parents or teachers as exasperatingly slow performance or failure to function in keeping with ability.

Anti-social behaviour in children and young adolescents sometimes displays a 'neurotic' quality which distinguishes it from the much commoner delinquent activities of the socially and emotionally deprived. For example episodes of stealing may be at the exclusive expense of one or both parents, often in such a manner as to invite discovery, the objects taken being sometimes worthless to the child. The appearance of obsessive or compulsive symptoms around the time of puberty in a previously healthy boy or girl should raise the possibility of a psychotic illness with atypical onset (pseudo-neurotic schizophrenia). Several months of close observation, not necessarily in hospital, however, may be required before a confident diagnosis emerges.

At the opposite extreme it must be noted that *rituals* are very common as transient behavioural features in otherwise healthy, well-functioning toddlers. As was mentioned in Chapter I these often occur at bed-time, and may amount to quite elaborate 'games' or tasks with precise sequence which must be identical at each performance, and often demand parent participation. In contrast to a neurosis, however, the child is developing well in other respects, is not anxiety-ridden, is given sufficient relief by the ritual to sleep soundly, and behaves normally the following day. Parents in such instances, should be advised to permit these common abnormalities of normal childhood and should be given the assurance that they are unlikely to persist longer than a few months. Even more commonplace in the young child is the expression of 'magical thinking' to ward off dangerous events. Many readers will recall the care to step clear of pavement cracks on the way to school, thereby ensuring good marks from the teacher! The rituals mentioned in chapter 9 as a characteristic feature of many autistic children tend to be elaborate and very persistent, but also serve to ward off anxiety.

Aetiology and prognosis of the neuroses

It is by no means certain what factors determine whether a child displays a transient stress-reaction or develops a neurotic illness. Organic disease or disability is unrelated directly to cause; the possibility of constitutional predisposition, as Freud recognized, is not so easily discarded, nor defined in any precise way. While there are many theoretical formulations, most share a general belief in the importance of early childhood experiences. Of late there has been a resurgence of the behaviourist viewpoint, neurotic disorder being viewed as maladaptive learning, so that inappropriate behaviour patterns become established. Logically, treatment procedures are designed to foster relearning of faulty patterns. *Behaviour therapy*, essentially a process of deconditioning, has had most success in monosymptomatic disorders.

Psychoanalytic theory seeks to explain the mental mechanisms which underlie neurotic symptomatology, and to modify these by interpretive psychotherapy. Most child psychiatric clinics provide individual or group techniques for the child in parallel with case-work interviews with the parents, or in selected cases, group sessions for the whole family. (See chapter 12) The rationale of these approaches is that the child has been subjected to attitudes and responses usually from the parents which in some important respect have undermined security, produced distorted perceptions or bewildering contradictions, as a result weakening instead of strengthening the child's coping mechanisms. All such psychodynamic therapies place central importance on the course of the relationship which develops between therapist and patient.

It has been demonstrated in at least one lengthy follow-up study into adulthood (Robins 1966) that the emotional disorders of neurotic type have a relatively benign prognosis in comparison with the conduct disorders.

Psycho-somatic disorders

Disorders which are characterized by definite abnormalities of

physiological function or organic structures
individuals are significantly influenced by
regards their onset, course, and prognosis a
or psychophysiologic. These disorders see
which are under the control of the autonom
the skin, respiratory, cerebrovascular, mus
the gastro-intestinal tract. Asthma, eczema
examples occuring commonly in all age-gr
It is widely recognized that in these illnesses there is no single cause
and that in different individuals, or even in the same individual at
different times allergy, infection, and psychological stress may be of
major significance. Another common example in childhood is
'periodic syndrome' including cyclical vomiting which may become
modified to migraine with increasing age. Peptic ulcer and ulcerative
colitis are less common before adulthood.

The psycho-somatic approach, which has become very popular
during the last quarter century especially in Western medicine, seeks
to bridge the artificial dichotomy between mind and body; to remind
us that a patient, child or adult, deserves to be considered not merely as
a multi-organ system but as a person. Flanders Dunbar (1946) one of
the pioneers of psycho-somatic medicine emphasized the patient's
'personality profile'. Others, especially of the psycho-analytic schools,
sought explanations in purely psychological events, especially in early
childhood, and in particular in the nature and quality of the parent-
child relationship. It is probably fair to say that none of these
hypotheses has proved entirely satisfactory, though the role of
emotional stress is generally accepted. In his classic monograph,
'Psycho-social Medicine', Halliday (1948) posed a cardinal question
when investigating such a patient. 'Why did this individual fall ill in
this particular way at this particular time?'. In every instance we have
to take into account: (1.) genetic make-up which determines the mode of
bodily response, for example, by an auto-immune reaction, (2.) environmental factors operating from birth onwards, whether infective,
traumatic, nutritional or psycho-social, and (3.) precipitants or
'triggers'.

The psychosomatic concomitants of childhood asthma have been
widely studied, and while it is frequently asserted that the asthmatic
child tends to be intelligent, anxious, and over-dependent, carefully
controlled studies, and especially where not restricted to hospital
populations, cast doubt on this stereotyped personality picture. Nor is
there convincing evidence for any one pattern of parent-child
interaction. It is not seriously in doubt, however, that emotional
factors can trigger an asthmatic attack. Moreover it is clear that long-

...e is significantly influenced by the way in which the ...ily copes with this chronic and often alarming illness. Pless ...kerton (1975) in a recent comprehensive review, reject the ...on that asthmatic children are a homogeneous group, either as ...gards personality characteristics or adaptation to the illness by themselves or their families. They contrast the child who shows an exaggerated 'invalid response' to relatively mild physical disability with the stoical boy or girl who consistently denies legitimate symptoms, and stress the crucial importance of appropriate counselling of child and parents where such discrepancies are identified. Purcell and his colleagues (1969) in a series of careful research studies have also identified subgroups of asthmatic children contrasting for example those who are 'steroid-dependent' and whose symptoms tend to persist after admission to hospital with those who remit rapidly in hospital, and who may again be subdivided into those whose attacks are primarily due to allergins with those 'triggered' by emotional factors. Family relationships, while significant as regards the child's adjustment, did not correlate with the severity of the asthma.

There has been much theorising and some careful investigation along psychosomatic lines into ulcerative colitis. While relatively rare in childhood, the course is often prolonged and debilitating. As with asthma, early investigators tried to identify a specific personality profile. For example Prugh (1951) emphasized the passive, dependent immature child, inhibited as regards any expression of aggressive impulses. But not all patients conform. A supposedly characteristic parental constellation, a domineering mother and an ineffectual father, has been described in association not only with ulcerative colitis but also with asthma and peptic ulcer. The evidence, however, is unconvincing. Moreover, few investigators have distinguished carefully between emotional factors antedating the illness and those reactive to prolonged pain and distress.

As regards peptic ulcer in childhood, by no means as rare as formerly believed, a familial tendency seems well-established. Here again claims have been made for particular patterns of disturbed parent-child relationship, but to date all that can be stated with confidence is that intra-familial stress, acute or chronic, is commonly encountered.

Wherever psychosomatic illness occurs in childhood we have to consider the impact of the illness itself on the family. The crude but popular notion that a child contrives to become ill in order 'to attract attention' does scant justice to the complexity of such situations. Being ill may fulfill the emotional need for a period of regression in a way that parent and society accepts, but if so we have to consider why this particular child does not have the possibility of occasional regressive episodes which are part of ordinary growing-up.

Often the symptom vanishes when the child is in hospital, only to recur on return home. As we have seen this *may* indicate relief from a stressful background. For some children, however, prolonged or repeated hospitalization itself contributes to emotional vulnerability which in turn may aggravate the presenting illness. The child's personality may therefore be a contributing factor to the psychosomatic problem, may be affected by the illness itself, by its impact on the family, or by the medical measures employed.

REFERENCES

Bowlby, J. (1972) *Attachment and Loss*. London: Hogarth.

Halliday, J.L. (1948) *Psycho-social Medicine*. London: Heinemann.

MacCarthy, D. & Boote, E.M. (1970) Parental rejection and stunting of growth. *Journal of Psychosomatic Research* 14, 259.

Prugh, D.J (1951) Influence of emotional factors on clinical course of ulcerative colitis in children. *Journal of Gastroenterology* 18, 339.

Psychopathological Disorders in Childhood (1968) New York: Group for Advancement of Psychiatry.

Purcell, K., Muser, L., Miklich, D., & Dietiker, K.E. (1969) Comparison of psychologic findings in variously defined asthmatic sub-groups. *Journal of Psychosomatic Research*, 13, 67.

Robins, L.N. (1966) *Deviant Children Grown Up*. Baltimore: Williams and Wilkins.

Spitz, R.A. (1946) Anaclitic depression. *Psychoanalytic Study of the Child*, 2, 313.

Winnicott, D.W. (1958) Transitional objects. In *Collected Papers*. London: Tavistock.

FURTHER READING

Freeman and Kaplan (eds.) (1967) Child psychiatry. In *Comprehensive Textbook of Psychiatry*. Baltimore: Williams and Wilkins.

Dunbar, H.F. (1946) *Emotions and Bodily Changes*. New York: Columbia.

Freud, A. (1965) *Normality and Pathology in Childhood*. London: Hogarth Press.

Pless, I.B. & Pinkerton, P. (1975) *Chronic Childhood Disorder-Promoting Patterns of Adjustment*. London: Henry Kimpton.

Prugh, D.A. (1963) Toward an understanding of psychosomatic concepts in relation to illness in children. In *Modern Perspectives in Child Development*. ed. Solnit. A.J. & Provence. S.A. New York: International Universities Press.

7

Developmental difficulties

Here we are concerned with children who for various reasons do not follow the usual developmental patterns. This is by no means a homogeneous group, and we shall consider them under three headings:
1. Children with developmental immaturity.
2. Children with special sensory handicaps.
3. Children with chronic physical illness or handicap.

1. CHILDREN WITH DEVELOPMENTAL IMMATURITY

In this group, although development follows the usual sequences, there is developmental delay, primarily affecting:
(a) Motor abilities.
(b) Spatial-perceptual skills.
(c) Speech.
These difficulties may occur in isolation or in various combinations. They may be present from birth, the result of immaturity rather than of brain damage.

(a) Motor

These children have difficulty in inhibiting unnecessary movements, poorly developed coordination, and usually poor muscle tone (Andre-Thomas and Saint-Anne-Dargassies, 1952). This hypotonicity may present as flat feet, knock-knees, excessive lumbar lordosis, protruding abdomen, or cubitus valgus. Deep reflexes may be exaggerated, without evidence of pyramidal tract lesions. Combined and alternating movements are poorly performed e.g. rapid pronation and supination of wrists. This *clumsy child syndrome*, as it is sometimes termed, is often associated with restlessness, hyperactivity and tics. Frustration-tolerance is low, and there tends to be poor emotional control.

The EEG is characterized by a high proportion of theta waves (5 to 7 cycles per second), posterior slow waves, and excessive reaction to hyperventilation. We regard this as a pattern of slow maturation rather than, as some have suggested, an inborn personality type or evidence of a brain lesion.

Environmental factors can significantly prolong a tendency to immaturity, and such children are among those mentioned in the chapter on aetiology who are vulnerable to emotional disturbances.

Hyperkinetic syndrome. Marked and persistent overactivity may, as we shall later discuss, be a feature of organic brain disease. Hyperactivity may also be a manifestation of anxiety, especially in the younger child. Thirdly, and what principally concerns us here, are these children who display marked overactivity from an early age, often noticed when they first begin to walk, and which is unrelated causally either to brain-damage or emotional disturbance. This is what is termed the 'hyperkinetic syndrome', and may be viewed as developmental delay in the progressive inhibition of motility and reactivity which takes place throughout the first seven or eight years of a child's life. At two to three years the hyperkinetic child is not only much more continuously active than the ordinary toddler but is markedly more distractible and talkative, and requires less sleep. Usually there is spontaneous gradual improvement, but the 'wear and tear' on family life, is considerable. Exclusion by nursery school is common. Secondary emotional disturbance is frequent, and this in turn may aggravate the presenting problem. Paradoxically small doses of dextro-amphetamine may be helpful, though it is essential that a close watch be kept on the use of a potentially habit-forming drug. Moreover the amphetamines may have side-effects such as poor appetite and sleep disturbance. Phenobarbitone tends in childhood to aggravate hyperactivity, and may even occasionally be its cause. Methylbenidate or butyrophenone. (Haloperidol) are preferable alternatives. (See Chapter 11.)

The hyperkinetic child may for a time require special day-care provision, and individual teaching in a distraction-free setting.

(b) Spatial-perceptual

Spatial orientation is a complex function involving the full integration of visual, auditory, and tactile stimuli. As well as developmental maturation, practice and training appear to play a part. For instance, African children reared along traditional lines have a better sense of spatial orientation than European children, or African children reared in a European fashion. (Biesheuvel, 1963.) Closely related is *laterality*, the expression of *cerebral dominance*. In the general population about 85 per cent are right-handed, 5 per cent left-handed, and the remaining 10 per cent show no clear-cut dominance. Of these a very few are truly ambidextrous; the remainder belong to the immature group, are equally clumsy with both hands, and have no definite lateral dominance. Spatial orientation is necessary for the mastery of reading, writing, and arithmetic. All these skills, however, also involve the capacity to decode symbols.

At the present time there is much controversy about children's difficulty in acquiring these skills. For example, some consider that there exists a specific reading disability of developmental origin with recognizable features amounting to a specific syndrome termed *dyslexia* (Critchley, 1964). Others are just as dogmatic that there is no such clinical entity, but that diverse factors, especially poor teaching techniques or interrupted schooling are the explanation of what they term *reading retardation*. It seems probable that both views are correct, but that developmental dyslexia accounts for a small minority of slow readers. (The older term 'congenital word blindness' is not recommended, as it implies the presence of a neurological disorder.) There is often the additional difficulty of poor spelling. Again this may be the result of an unsatisfactory learning experience (and in the case of English idiosyncrasies of the language), or in some children great difficulty in distinguishing symmetrical letters such as 'p' and 'q', or 'b' and 'd'. Letters may also be placed out of sequence e.g. 'prat' instead of 'part'. It is not clear why severe reading retardation is so often found in association with conduct disorder (delinquency).

Some children spontaneously write from right to left, so called *mirror-writing*. This is a common transient feature during the first years of schooling. It is probably more frequent in left-handed children, and may be a reason for trying to persuade the child to use the right hand. Such a decision must always be made very carefully on the advice of an educational psychologist or other competent specialist. Formerly it was considered a disability to be left-handed, and this was counteracted with diligence, often misguidedly, though there is no truth in the widely-held belief that this is a cause of stuttering. Slowness or difficulty in writing may of course, be the result of clumsiness, a pencil *dyspraxia*.

In the common varieties of reading disability the child, given encouragement and skilled educational help usually learns to read in time, but may not become fluent till a relatively late age, and may never read for pleasure. It can be readily understood that such children may acquire considerable problems of adjustment both at home and at school. They may be regarded as 'lazy pupils', may be regularly punished without benefit, and may understandably acquire a persistently negative attitude to all educational approaches. The sensitive, skilled management of these problems is not only frequently rewarded by educational progress, but can make a significant contribution to the emotional well-being of the child and his family.

(c) Developmental speech lag

In the young child this often presents a challenging diagnostic exercise. There is some evidence that slow speech development may occur in isolation i.e. in a child of ordinary intellectual endowment, with unimpaired hearing and intact neural and vocal apparatus. There is a familial tendency, and males are chiefly affected. These boys eventually achieve ordinary speech development but are slow starters. While a family history may be suggestive, it is essential to exclude mental handicap or deafness, in the first year of life if possible. Emotional deprivation, and inadequate or confusing auditory stimulation may also interfere with speech development, e.g. the over protected or infantilized child, or the child reared in a non-speaking environment, for example by deaf-mute parents. Twins are sometimes observed to develop a private communication system using an extensive sign language and an esoteric jargon. *Elective mutism* is a purely psychological disturbance in which the child talks to a very limited number of persons, often the mother only, and is completely silent in all other situations. The degree of emotional disturbance may be slight and transient, or may amount to a severe personality disorder. Rarer causes of delayed or abnormal speech are early childhood autism, (discussed in chapter 9) and *congenital dysphasia* with impaired language comprehension. To such a child ordinary conversation is perceived as a series of meaningless sounds.

2.   CHILDREN WITH SPECIAL SENSORY HANDICAPS

(a) Visual impairment

Because of the common embryological origin of the brain and the eye there is sometimes combined impairment. With careful examination blindness can be diagnosed even in the young infant. The presence of a pupillary light reaction is by no means absolute evidence of sight. The blind infant does not follow with his eyes at the age of 2 to 3 months and there may also be abnormal movements of the eyeballs or in contrast an abnormal lack of motility. Blind children also frequently develop stereotypies such as rubbing the eyeballs, probably producing visual sensations of an elementary type. Obviously the earlier the diagnosis of blindness is made the better. The intelligent blind child can learn to read *braille* and have a normal scholastic career. In infancy it is quite easy to misdiagnose blindness for mental retardation or even childhood autism.

Important also is the poor-sighted child. In infancy it may be thought that there is complete blindness when actually there is delayed myelination of the optic nerve. It is clear therefore that this kind of assessment calls for a paediatric ophthalmologist. The young child with imperfect vision should be helped as early as possible with suitable spectacles though it may not be easy to prescribe the appropriate lenses.

The visually handicapped child should ordinarily be in a normal school setting. If necessary he may join a special class, but as a rule unless there is no other solution, the blind or partially sighted child should not be removed from home, being more prone than normal children to the effects of emotional deprivation. We occasionally encounter an infant whose blindness is due to bilateral congenital cataract which can be cured by surgery. It is important that this should be done in the early months of life, as late acquisition of vision may result in severe psychiatric disturbance.

(b) Hearing impairment
Deafness can be inherited. It can also be produced by rubella infection during pregnancy, or later in life by a toxic agent such as streptomycin or mumps virus.

As in the case of visual handicap early diagnosis of hearing loss is important and difficult. Infants may be deaf as far as ordinary conversational frequencies are concerned (between 2000 and 4000hz) but can hear sounds belonging to other ranges of frequency. In testing the young infant the human voice and a range of sounding toys can be used. The diagnositic reliability of conditioning reflexes is a controversial matter. Between the ages of 2 and 4 years the 'peep show' techniques can be used; after the age of 4 years classical audiometry becomes possible. Deaf and hard-of-hearing children are prone to behaviour difficulties. In the face of emotional stress there may be retreat into unresponsiveness even an autistic type of withdrawal, and as with the deaf adult there is sometimes a tendency to over-suspiciousness.

(c) Congenital indifference to pain
This is a very rare and poorly understood condition. These children seem insensitive to pain, and as a result may sustain repeated burns or other injuries. No neuro-anatomical localization has been identified. Some are probably genetically determined.

3. CHILDREN WITH CHRONIC PHYSICAL ILLNESSES AND HANDICAPS

Chronic physical illness or handicap may have effects on social and emotional development and educational progress. Repeated or prolonged hospitalization for whatever reason is liable to disrupt ties with parents, home, sibs and peer group unless physicians and surgeons are constantly alert to the need for regular and frequent visiting by parents, and to the possibility of home or day-hospital care whenever practical. Where there is marked restriction of movement because of surgical appliances, paralysis, or cardiorespiratory dysfunction, imaginative play and occupational programmes geared to the child's developmental level can do much to compensate. Every paediatric unit should have a hospital school not only to prevent long interruptions in education, but to sustain intellectual stimulation, as well as maintaining links with the outside world. We must not underestimate the importance for the hospitalized child of continuity of personal contact by nurses, teachers, and play-leaders, as well as the activities themselves. Children with disabling physical handicaps will often require to attend special day classes or schools. Those with minor disabilities will usually gain immeasurably from attendance at an ordinary school.

The emotional climate of the family can be predominantly overprotective, rejecting, or fluctuate widely and inconsistently. In many medical conditions life expectancy is improving. Children with chronic renal disease or leukaemia for example may survive for years. In such circumstances anxiety is inescapable for both parents and child, though it may be expressed deviously e.g. by naughtiness or more often a bland conformity in a child; by indulgence or irascibility in a parent. In conditions like severe poliomyelitis with extensive paralysis, children often develop compensatory phantasies. The haemophiliac may become timid and passive, or by contrast, defiantly daring and active. When relationships with medical or nursing staff, or for that matter with parents are poor, the severely dyspnoeic child is liable to indulge in strenuous exertion, the diabetic child in overeating, the epileptic child to 'forget' to take his anticonvulsants.

Finally we have to consider the care of the dying child, especially when the expectation of life though limited, is of uncertain duration. The facts of the situation have to be presented to the parents, a task which usually falls to the paediatrician or to the family doctor. Each interview is a very individual matter, for which there can be no hard and fast rules beyond the obvious ones of reasonable time and privacy. A particularly difficult question is what, if anything, should be said to the child. Of course, not only ill children ask questions about death and dying. Even in the third or fourth year of life there is curiosity about relatives such as grandparents, who are no longer visible. Many parents use the traditional formula 'They've gone to Heaven', and then have to cope with a succession of perfectly logical questions, such as 'When will they be coming back?', 'Can we go and visit?' What we so often ignore, however, is that even very young children can be extremely perceptive about how we, the adults, are reacting to the situation ourselves. Thus we return to the familiar theme, that how we behave is often as significant for the child as what we say.

With regard to death, as with all other emotionally important happenings, the notion that children are too young to understand or to notice is probably best discarded after infancy.

In the ward situation, children likewise take their cues from doctors and nurses. If there is an atmosphere of informal communication between patients and staff, then the child will ask searching questions. Discretion is needed in replying to questions about the death of another patient, or about the nature of their own illness, and all staff need to share ideas about how to respond. If this whole issue is ignored, as if by so doing it would somehow cease to exist, the children often direct their anxious questions to orderlies or ward-maids who may or may not react appropriately. Young and inexperienced medical and nursing staff need help in coping with death and dying in a way which allows them to use personal resources of sympathy and intuition in a constructive manner.

Families invariably need support after a bereavement, especially perhaps when the death is that of a child. Some turn to traditional religious observance and welcome the guidance and support of their spiritual leader. The physician is often best placed to detect those who are likely to require the help of a psychiatric social-worker. Occasionally a bereavement reaction, instead of progressing from the phase of mourning to steady recovery, merges insidiously into a depressive state calling for psychiatric treatment. It is important also to be on the alert for the signs of inappropriate reaction to a bereavement.

A temporary phase of emotional denial is common but if persistent should be regarded as a psychological danger signal.

REFERENCES
André-Thomas and Saint-Anne-Dargassies (1952) *Etudes Neurologiques sur le Nouveau-né et le jeune Nourrisson*, Paris: Masson & Perrin.
Biesheuvel, S. (1963). The growth of abilities and character in Symposium on current problems in the behavioural sciences in South Africa. *South African Journal of Science* 59, (8), 375–368.
Critchley, M. (1964) *Developmental Dyslexia*. London: Heinemann.

FURTHER READING
Anthony, E. J. and Koupernik, C. (Eds.) (1973) *The Child in his Family*. Vol. 2. New York: Wiley.
Rutter, M., Tizard, J. and Whitmore, K. (1970) *Education, Health and Behaviour*. London: Longman.
Touwen, B. C. L. and Prechtl, H.F.R. (1970) The neurological examination of the child with minor nervous dysfunction. *Clinics in Developmental Medicine No. 38.* London, Heinemann; and Philadelphia, Lipincott.

8

Personality disorders and borderline states

Personality disorders are characterized by fixed traits affecting the behaviour, attitude, modes of thinking and reactions of the individual. In contrast to the neuroses there is neither psychic conflict nor necessarily any anxiety. We are in danger, however, of presenting an oversimplified dichotomy; on the one hand the personality disorders, which were formerly regarded as invariably constitutional in origin, and on the other, the neuroses, the result of inadequate adjustment to the environment. It would be truer to say that personality in the sense of the style of the individual, involving as it does the individual's mode of reaction to a variety of situations, manner of relating to other people, and coping mechanisms under stress, is the product of inherited constitutional factors and life experience. An abnormal personality may result from an organic insult to the central nervous system; it is also now well established, however, that similar if not identical results may be a sequel to abnormal influences, especially in the early stages of childhood. It would seem therefore at the present stage of our knowledge that a child whose biological equipment is fragile will tend to suffer permanent effects from unfavourable influences arising in the psychological milieu.

Numerous categories have been described under the general headings of 'personality disorder' but rather than list these we prefer to present a continuum with a rather characteristic and contrasting clinical picture at either extremity. At the one end we find compulsive, rigidly organized personalities who in a particular context, for instance in war time, prove to be very 'well adjusted'. In peace time these same individuals may have considerable social problems, often tending to adjust well to an authoritarian type of regime, but poorly to an open competitive society. At the other end of the continuum are those dysharmonic personalities with a very narrow margin of adjustment who tend to display marked impulsiveness with a propensity for 'acting out', in a manner which is unacceptable to our society.

For descriptive purposes we identify two main groups of personality disorders:

I.   Those presenting various types of personality organization.
II.   Those who fail to abide by the mores of society.

Group I

1. *Obsessive compulsive personality*. This describes a tightly organized, very orderly individual who tends when there is conflict to change his or her environment. The social behaviour of this type of person is very close to that of the classical paranoiac or paranoid personality type. It also corresponds to the 'anal' personality which Freud considered to be due to a fixation or hold-up at a development level corresponding to the stage of achievement of sphincter control. With extreme degrees of such rigidity the picture merges with that of the 'borderline' psychotic.

2. In contrast there is the *hysterical personality* which is as flexible as the other is rigid, as suggestible as the other is not. Obsessional personalities in a sense are overmature; hysterical personalities childish. In the latter, early environment often seems to play an important causal role. Whereas some such individuals have lacked affection in the early stages others have been overprotected—though admittedly this often conceals relative deprivation. One can not confidently assume aetiology from personality type. Obsessional and hysterical personalities may be contrasted in yet another way; the former are very much the introverts, the latter the extraverts, in the terminology of Jung. Actually the Jungian concept is of a continuum from introversion to extroversion, meaning that each individual is to a lesser or greater extent mainly concerned with the inner or the outer world.

As with the neuroses we have to be particularly cautious as far as children are concerned in delineating personality types. Many of the features of ordinary early childhood behaviour and attitudes are close to what we have described as hysterical personality, for example the inconsistency, the tendency to manipulate the environment, to dramatize. It is also common for a young child to speak aloud his phantasy.

3. The *seclusive personality* is introverted, happy to be alone, often immersed in day-dreaming but at the same time capable of excellent functioning especially in the field of abstract thought. It has been suggested that such individuals are schizoid and prone to develop schizophrenia but it is doubtful whether there is sufficient evidence for this view.

4. *Psychopathic personality* or *sociopathic personality* (see group II). This category is characterized by the violence of tension and of discharge. Some individuals of this type have strong aggressive drives

while their moral or social inhibitions are poorly developed; others by contrast present a type of neurotic repetitive behaviour which tends to have some symbolic meaning, and represents an endless struggle between drive and prohibition. Identical behaviour may have quite different prognostic implications. The behaviour pattern itself, however apparently serious, for example fire-setting or car-thieving, may be symptomatic of a transient emotional conflict or of an established dysharmonic personality. The fate of such individuals depends on the way society treats them and is willing to accept them. It is important to note the role of the environment in the fate of such personalities. For instance in the case of adolescents a tendency to alcohol indulgence, drug addiction, or membership of a gang may all lead to delinquency; in war time they may be heroes. It is worth recalling the comment of Bovet (1951) that delinquency is not a medical or psychiatric concept but a legal one.

Group II

Here we are concerned with a different set of criteria namely that of adjustment or opposition to generally accepted moral standards in a given social group. Clearly the stage of development of the child or adolescent has to be taken carefully into account as regards such behaviour patterns as lying, stealing, aggression or other antisocial traits.

1. *Sociopathic personality* (corresponding to type (4) in the first group). Persistently aggressive, sadistic, even murderous behaviour is encountered from time to time even in early childhood. Sometimes there is evidence of a brain lesion, especially a temporal lobe focus. One of us (CK) had an opportunity to observe a 10-year-old child who, following partial recovery from tuberculous meningitis with resultant lesions in the basal region of the brain and calcification visible on X-ray, had become a very real danger to small children and animals. Occasionally such behaviour is witnessed in psychotic children.

Sometimes we do not find evidence of any organic lesion of the central nervous system or of psychosis. In the majority of these the causal factor is severe emotional deprivation of the type described by Bowlby (1952), resulting in the development of an *affectionless character* which may progress to adult *sociopathy*. Some of these children have had prolonged separation experiences in the first few years, while others have been cared for by a succession of mother figures. In some instances the mother has lacked the capacity to give care and affection. Not all children succumb even to these experiences but clearly a proportion do. It is well to remember, however, that the normality or otherwise of behaviour traits have to be seen in a particular cultural context. For instance Margaret Mead (1935) in a well-known essay compares the gentle Arapesh who are reared in a climate of mutual love, trust, and confidence, and in contrast the hard violent Mundugumor who regard distrust and aggression as desirable traits from childhood onwards.

2. *Sexual deviations.*

(i) Occasionally very young children, even infants, may be observed to indulge in a frantic type of masturbation far beyond anything that is ordinarily present. Some such children are mentally retarded, others are autistic, and still others having been deprived of affection and care in their early lives resort to their own bodies for satisfaction. Some children have been the victims of seduction and premature stimulation by other children or adults. Instances have been recorded where this has happened to the offspring of prostitutes at the hands of their patrons. The whole question of masturbation has to be put in perspective. During the puritanical Victorian era there were widely held fears about the possible dire consequences of masturbation, which it was widely believed could lead to disease, insanity or sterility, ideas quite without foundation. Nevertheless, it is equally untrue that all masturbation can be ignored as irrelevant by the clinician. Where it is persistent and especially where there is no concern for ordinary modesty it is an indication for assessment of the child's overall emotional development.

(ii) Effeminacy in boys. This refers not only to sexual development as such, but to general behaviour and attitudes, interest in games, and choice of company. Such boys tend to avoid fighting, and to be markedly passive. It is a pattern which sometimes develops later into male homosexuality. Commonly there has been a very close relationship with the mother and remote one with the father, but it is by no means clear whether the overprotective maternal relationship is an unconscious response on the mother's part to this type of son rather than being its cause. The origins of homosexuality in both sexes are as yet quite unclear. Now that the subject is no longer taboo serious researches are being undertaken into the origin of both male and female homosexuality. It is unlikely that seduction of a child by an adult of the same sex of itself causes sexual deviance, but it may well happen that when the tendency is already there an experience of this kind can deflect sexual orientation towards homosexuality. It is very important that the psychiatrist should distinguish between homosexuality, which is not strictly speaking treatable, although the individual may be greatly helped in adjusting to his or her sexual orientation, and the neurotic fear of being homosexual which is a variety of phobia calling for psychotherapy with reasonable hope of success.

(iii) Childhood transvestism. In boys even before puberty intense sexual stimulation is sometimes obtained by wearing feminine dress and underwear. This behaviour is usually a stimulus to masturbation phantasies. Minor transvestism is quite common among adults and is completely compatible with an ordinary satisfying heterosexual adjustment. Bizarre forms which interfere with ordinary life activities tend to be associated with complex personality problems and are not very responsive to any known forms of treatment. We have previously noted that transitory homosexual phases may be present in both sexes, both before and after puberty. Boys and girls reared in single sex communities such as boarding schools are likely to have even stronger tendencies in this direction, but this is by no means always the precursor of a persistent homosexual orientation.

BORDERLINE STATES

This term describes the group of disorders which lie between the neuroses and the psychoses. The symptomatology is similar to that of the neuroses but the severity is much greater. Although thought disorder is not manifest, reality testing is weakened and at moments of crisis may temporarily disintegrate. The following three examples will serve to illustrate these borderline states:

1. Severe obsessional states. These make their appearance in later childhood and during adolescence, and may be so intense that they can completely interfere with a normal way of life. Guilt feelings, the permanent conviction of sinning are common; affected children may constantly accuse themselves of having been responsible by their thoughts alone for the illness or death of someone near to them. Or there may be the persistent anxiety of being poisoned. A common finding in such individuals is unresolved aggression. Whereas in the first instance the individual fears his own impulses, these are later projected on to the outer world. The resultant fear of retribution leads to further symptom-formation.

Of a variety of severe obsessional states the most peculiar is perhaps the syndrome of Gilles de la Tourette. In this condition, which is occasionally observed in children and adolescents, multiple and refractory tics accompany the involuntary utterance of obscene words and phrases. It is by no means certain that this is a definite syndrome, and its aetiology is unknown. Improvement has been obtained with butyrophenones (Haloperidol), and a few cases have recently been submitted to neurosurgical procedures with as yet uncertain long-term results.

In all these severe obsessional states the prognosis must be guarded.

They may disappear for a time but have a tendency to recur. Occasionally they are symptomatic of schizophrenia. Improvement may occasionally permit of ordinary social life, the resulting state being similar to the obsessional personality previously described.

2. Anorexia nervosa. This disorder is encountered almost exclusively in girls, male cases amounting to no more than one in twenty. Usually the onset is related to a tendency to slight or moderate overweight, and as a result of teasing or anxiety about weight, the girls embark on a reducing diet. Strictly speaking 'anorexia' is not really an appropriate description at this stage as these girls refrain from eating although they have a good appetite and have to struggle to resist it. The two main symptoms soon appear, namely, rapid and intense loss of weight, and amenorrhoea. With the severe loss of weight a true anorexia rapidly develops. In spite of this there is often marked brightness and overactivity. Invariably the family circle becomes anxious and all sorts of techniques are used to induce eating. At one time it was thought that there might be some obscure endocrine or neurological basis for anorexia nervosa, but it is now recognized that this is a psychiatric disorder and that the associated physical symptoms are entirely the consequences of weight loss and dietary disequilibrium. Gain in weight can often be achieved only when the girl is isolated from the family. Management calls for considerable skill on the part of medical and perhaps especially nursing staff. It is usually possible to obtain improvement without severely coercive feeding methods, sometimes with the assistance of tranquillization. Relapses are common, and although about 50 per cent are finally cured, about another quarter have residual neurotic symptoms often related to food and feeding. A few progress to overeating and obesity. A small proportion especially in affected males eventually develop typical features of schizophrenia. It is difficult to place anorexia nervosa confidently in any particular psychiatric category. Some show resemblances to an hysterical picture, some to a severe obsessional state, others are decidedly depressive in mood, and a few as we have seen proceed to schizophrenia. It is on account of this uncertain course that we place them among the borderline states.

3. Dysmorphophobia. This refers to a condition in which a child or adolescent rejects some aspect of the body, occasionally becoming delusional. The preoccupation is usually with some part of the face, often the nose, sometimes the eyes, the ears or the mouth. Girls are often concerned about the shape of the breasts, boys about the size of the external genitalia. It is hardly surprising that these concerns tend to be frequent during adolescence, this being a time when the body undergoes marked changes both of structure and function, in

particular the acquisition of secondary sexual characteristics. And of course attraction towards and by the opposite sex is closely bound up with bodily appearance. Common is the conviction of being constantly under scrutiny by other people, and the belief in an imperfection of this kind may often lead to shyness, seclusion or occasionally aggressiveness. In instances where there are persistent requests for plastic surgical procedures a psychiatric opinion is usually advisable. In the more severely obsessed or intermittently delusional individual no procedure is likely to prove satisfactory. Closely related are the anxieties quite often encountered among adolescents that the body emits an unpleasant odour. All or any of these delusional ideas have been known to result in suicide.

Personality disorders and borderline states have a special importance in child psychiatry in that, occurring in parents or near relatives, these may be important causal factors in the development of emotional difficulties in the child. The implications of this for aetiology and treatment will be considered further in the chapter on family psychiatry.

REFERENCES

Bovet, L. (1951) *Psychiatric Aspects of Juvenile Delinquency*. W.H.O. Monograph I.
Bowlby, J. (1952) *Maternal Care and Mental Health*. W.H.O. Monograph Series No. 2.
Mead, M. (1935) *Sex and Temperament in Three Primitive Societies*. New York: Mentor.

FURTHER READING

Bruce, H. (1974) *Eating Disorders* London: Routledge and Kegan Paul.
Crisp, A. H. (1965) Some aspects of the evolution, presentation, and follow-up of anorexia nervosa. *Proceedings of the Royal Society of Medicine*, 58, 814.
Geleerd, E. R. (1958) Borderline states in childhood and adolescence. *Psychoanalytic Study of the Child* 13, 279–295.
Schneider, K. (1958) *Psychopathic Personalities*. London: Cassell.

9

Psychotic and autistic states

Psychosis is a general term meaning a continuously bizarre and unpredictable pattern of behaviour. In childhood two main clinical syndromes may be differentiated:
1. Early Infantile Autism, first described by Kanner (1943), and
2. Childhood Schizophrenia, or what Kolvin (1971) has termed Late Onset Psychosis.

Early childhood autism. Autism means withdrawal, referring to the central feature, a non-relatedness to other people, which although often not noticed at the time is probably always present from infancy. Speech development is invariably affected, and this in addition to the withdrawn state makes examination, psychiatric or psychometric, extremely difficult.

Kanner (1943) in his original description noted a further characteristic, what he called 'an obsessional desire for sameness'. We shall consider these features in some detail.

Withdrawal or autism. These children do not make normal contact with others. They may pay no attention whatsoever when spoken to, yet the fact that they can reproduce accurately phrases or snatches of song shows that they are not deaf. Parents explain that they 'can't get through', that the child makes them feel 'like a piece of furniture, as if the didn't exist'. Ordinary eye-to-eye contact is lacking. With direct questioning we sometimes learn that their extraordinarily 'good' behaviour as babies really amounted to self-absorption. Parents recall how the infant would sit quietly for long periods 'playing' with his hands, examining the pram-covers, gazing up at trees. This *preoccupation with objects* becomes more striking as the child becomes older, when there is an apparent fascination with wheels, shiny surfaces, or anything mechanical.

Abnormalities of speech. The child may occasionally remain mute. More often words appear at the usual time, but at around 18 months to 2 years these small achievements may be lost. Characteristically there is a marked tendency to repeat a phrase or word exactly as spoken (*echolalia*). Pronouns cause trouble, 'you' and 'I' often seemingly being confused. These children often refer to themselves as 'you', 'he' or 'she'. Even where speech is relatively well developed it often has a rather stilted quality, with slight oddities of syntax, monotony of expression, and a rather extreme literalness. If spoken to figuratively an autistic child may reply quaintly. When asked to 'draw a picture', he may do just that, frame and all! A father who complained that his child's questions would make him 'climb the wall' was asked with genuine curiosity how he would avoid falling down.

Obsessional desire for sameness. Autistic children become distressed, often acutely so, if some accustomed pattern is upset. It may be their daily routine, the arrangement of books in a cupboard, or the route taken on a familiar journey. They are inconsolable till the 'sameness' is restored. Though there is seldom much interest in toys as such there is often a seeming fascination with wheels, spinning toys, pieces of string, sand and water, and light and shade. Ordinary household articles such as clothes-pegs, match-boxes, and milk-bottle tops may provide material for absorbed pattern-making. Often elaborate arrangements are painstakingly produced, and here also any interruption of the activity or disarrangement of the patterns can provoke marked distress. The ability to reproduce exactly such complex designs is evidence of a special kind of memory. Television commercials, the wording on advertisement hoardings, the theme from a symphony, may all be reproduced with perfect if mechanical accuracy.

Unusual postures and movements are also commonly present. The child may twirl or rock monotonously, or place the hands in unusual positions and seem to examine them closely. The hands are often clapped over the ears, and walking may be on tip-toe. Though occasionally encountered in association with blindness or deafness, the autistic child usually has intact hearing and vision. It is not difficult to appreciate that quite often the condition is mistaken for deafness, mental handicap, or both. While audiometric examination may be sabotaged by the child's intense interest in the apparatus and total disregard of the examiner, the sudden production of a complex phrase or snatch of music effectively rules out deafness. Psychological testing can sometimes give useful hints of ability by using non-verbal items. There are often considerable intellectual deficits.

Physical examination is usually quite negative. No neurological process or biochemical abnormality has been detected though about twenty per cent develop convulsions in later life. Early infantile autism is unrelated to adult-type schizophrenia. It is unlikely that autism can be produced by environmental factors alone. What has been described as 'mechanical', detached mothering is not the sole cause of the autistic state, though it may occasionally be the maternal reaction to an unresponsive baby. The disorder is probably present from birth though its precise cause remains unknown. It can not be explained solely on the basis of a developmental language disorder though comprehension of the spoken word is often imperfect.

Psychotherapy for the young autistic child has a useful place in selected cases. With skill and good fortune the therapist may gain an understanding of the child's pathological anxieties for example about close physical contact, certain types of noise, ordinary bodily functions such as breathing, laughing, urinating and so on. With safe repetition and reassurance the child can sometimes be helped to discard the exaggerated 'defences' which appear whenever there is anxiety e.g. complex rituals. Equally important, the therapist can 'interpret' the child's behaviour and special needs to the parents, being supportive but not judgemental. Common-sense management is of no avail whatsoever with autistic children. It makes matters worse, moreover, when the parents are convinced, as they so often are, that they have been responsible for the child's condition. Drugs provide no more than symptomatic relief of for example overactivity or insomnia.

Doctors need to know that these unusual patients may have difficulty in localizing pain, and can be extremely distressed and hard to manage if away from familiar places and persons. If hospitalization is needed for medical or surgical reasons, facilities should be sought which allow the mother to be admitted also.

The stress of living with such a child is great on both parents and siblings. There is need for knowledgeable and skilled counselling, day-care facilities with trained staff, and frequent short-term residential care to allow the family to have a respite. Such resources are still very limited in numbers and facilities. Even less available are hospitals or other child psychiatric units able to care adequately for autistic children in long-term residential care. It is very unusual for there to be more than one autistic child in a family.

The prognosis varies. Kanner recognized that it was significantly worse if by the age of 5 years the child was still mute. In such cases long-term residential care may be required, and the final level of social and intellectual competence very poor. At the other extreme, the child may be able to attend day-school though usually a good deal of individual or at most small-group teaching is required. The adult picture tends to be that of a very shy, nervous, somewhat odd individual who tends to avoid company but may be reasonably proficient in an occupation which is not too demanding of initiative or flexibility.

CHILDHOOD SCHIZOPHRENIA

Here the onset tends to be insidious, odd behaviour being observable sometimes for years before one can identify clear-cut psychotic signs such as hallucinations, delusions, blocking of thought, blunting of emotion, or abnormalities of mood. Stereotyped movements, rituals, and obsessional traits are all common. Although such children do not maintain lasting social relationships, this is not because they are 'autistic' but rather because their unpredictable, chaotic, wildly unconventional behaviour is upsetting, even frightening to other children, and indeed to adults. The prognosis in childhood schizophrenia while always guarded, tends to be better the more acute the onset. Tranquillizers of the phenothiazine group are sometimes rapidly effective. Intelligence varies, but is commonly below average.

Autistic and schizophrenic disorders of childhood all require specialized child psychiatric facilities for assessment, and many for management and long-term support. Some of the main contrasting features between early infantile autism and childhood schizophrenia are summarized in Table 1. Schizophrenia rarely begins before late adolescence or early adult life.

Both of these syndromes are rare, but it is not uncommon for severe mental handicap to be accompanied by autistic or psychotic-like behaviour.

DEPRESSION

Endogenous depression occurs very rarely in childhood. Depressive symptoms may, however, predominate in the early stages of schizophrenia, for example in adolescence. Transient episodes of depression sometimes with suicidal preoccupation are also common at

Table 1

	Early infantile autism	Childhood schizophrenia
Onset	From birth	From early childhood
Hallucinations and delusions	Absent	Commonly present
Prevalence of schizophrenia in relatives	Not raised	Above that of controls
Socio-economic class of parents	Tends to be high	Tends to be low
Response to phenothiazines	Very poor	Good or fair

this stage as prominent symptoms of an adolescent crisis. As was mentioned in the discussion of the neuroses, reactive or neurotic depression is quite common in early life, and often presents with either psychosomatic features or educational difficulties.

Finally, a psychotic syndrome may occur as a *symptomatic psychosis*, secondary to progressive neurological disease, to infection, or as a toxic reaction to drugs such as LSD, amphetamine, or occasionally cortico-steroids.

REFERENCES

Kanner, L. (1943) Autistic disturbances of affective contact. *Nervous Child*, **2**, 217.

Kolvin, I. (1971) Studies in the childhood psychoses. *British Journal of Psychiatry* **118**, 381.

FURTHER READING

Coppen, A. and Walk, A. (eds.) (1967) *Recent Developments in Schizophrenia*. R.M.P.A. London: Invicta.

Creak, M. *et al.*, (1964) Schizophrenic syndrome in childhood. *Developmental Medicine and Child Neurology*, **4**, (6), 530-535.

Rutter, M. (ed.) (1971) *Infantile Autism: Concepts, Characteristics and Treatment*. Edinburgh: Churchill Livingstone.

Stone, F.H. (1970) The autistic child. *Practitioner*, **205**, 313-318.

Wing, L. (1971) *Autistic Children*. London: Constable.

10

Brain syndromes

BRAIN SYNDROMES AND EMOTIONAL DISORDER

In this chapter we shall consider the relationship between psychiatric disorders of childhood and organic disease of the brain. As we previously discussed in the chapter on aetiology the majority of reactive or stress disorders, as well as the neuroses and many personality disorders are social and/or psychological in origin. In such cases the presence of brain pathology may be fortuitous, or may have contributed to aetiology although not of itself the sole, or direct cause. We also raised the question of 'vulnerability' to emotional disorder, and noted that children with brain syndromes are more than ordinarily vulnerable to all forms of environmental stress; children with physical handicaps, but intact nervous systems, are also 'vulnerable' to stress, but much less markedly so (Rutter, 1969).

Further, many children with brain syndromes show no evidence of psychiatric illness nor indeed of significant emotional disturbance. So, with limited exceptions, the relationship between brain pathology and psychopathology is indirect.

An interesting problem is posed by children who after sustaining a head injury develop behaviour difficulties, either for the first time or in markedly exacerbated form. Occasionally this is the direct outcome of localized cerebral damage. Commonly however, the injury has been slight, for example mild concussion without residual neurological signs, but a background inquiry reveals long-standing familial stress. The accident appears to act as a 'trigger' for latent psychopathology.

We have to bear in mind always the reaction of parents, family, school, and community to a child with a brain syndrome, whether this is apparent as in cerebral palsy, or 'invisible' as in epilepsy. For many lay people it is much easier to feel sympathetic towards an obviously handicapped child even if they are slow to progress and to learn, than towards an apparently healthy child with inexplicable episodes of difficult behaviour, and perhaps occasional frightening 'turns'.

The cause of the organic damage often dates from the antenatal, perinatal period, or early months of life. It is here that the opportunities for prevention are most promising in particular the care of the pregnant woman, the prevention and treatment of toxaemia, and careful obstetric management.

Criteria and diagnosis

Firstly there may be aetiological evidence of cerebral damage having occurred at a prenatal, perinatal or postnatal stage of development. This may be traumatic, infective, metabolic or toxic in origin. There may be an inborn error of metabolism such as phenylketonuria or galactosaemia. It may be due to genetic transmission as in the lipoidosis, tuberose sclerosis, muscular dystrophy, or Friedreich's ataxia. Or it may be associated with a chromosomal abnormality as in Down's syndrome.

Secondly there may be clinical evidence. Physical examination may reveal the presence of neurological signs. There may be abnormal appearances in the electroencephalogram, confirmatory evidence from pneumoencephalography, echography, arteriography or scanning. Epileptic seizures are of themselves evidence of brain dysfunction. However, we should note that non-specific abnormalities are often present in the EEG of children with emotional disorders of psychological origin.

Thirdly there is the more controversial issue of psychological and psychiatric evidence. Many clinicians accept that the association of disorders of orientation in time and space, of learning abilities, memory, language and other cognitive functioning suggest alteration in brain function. Sometimes the clinical picture is less obvious, the symptomatology more subtle. Some children for example are hyperkinetic, have unexplained mood disorders, depressive or manic; others are violent and aggressive or may have a very localized impairment of intellectual functioning. Some severe dyslexias are probably organic in origin. Psychological tests may reveal discrepancies between verbal and performance skills, difficulties with spatial orientation or with symbolic thinking.

To some clinicians all of these findings are 'soft signs' and are therefore not acceptable as unequivocal evidence of neurological damage or impairment. We take the view that a combination of reliable medical and psychosocial history plus the clinical features of the type we have described may be more valuable than orthodox neurological examination. Emotional disturbance in a brain-damaged child may take the form of a stress reaction, a neurosis, a personality disorder, or occasionally a psychotic state. Moreover, the severity of the emotional disturbance, as we have already discussed is determined by many factors of which the degree of organic brain impairment is only one.

ACUTE CEREBRAL SYNDROMES

These may be infective, toxic, allergic, metabolic, or traumatic. The infection may be bacterial or viral causing inflammation of the brain and/or the meninges. Encephalitis may be difficult to diagnose with certainty, but the clinician will particularly note disturbances of consciousness, hyperpyrexia, abnormalities in the cerebrospinal fluid, and profound changes in the electroencephalogram. Sometimes, however, the diagnosis is made only retrospectively. Common toxic agents in childhood are substances swallowed by accident such as atropine, tricyclic antidepressants, and other psychotropic drugs. Occasionally lead poisoning may produce brain-damage. Rarer causes are alcohol, industrial and domestic fluids, and in recent times psychedelic drugs. The third important cause of acute cerebral injury in childhood is trauma, the result of falls, road accidents, or child abuse. Impulsive, overactive, or retarded children are particularly accident-prone, so that brain-damage may be cumulative. The following example illustrates the way in which an acute brain syndrome may be present with psychiatric features. A boy of 14 years previously a satisfactory pupil was referred to a department of child psychiatry because of poor school-work. There was a noticeable deterioration in writing, with a tendency to misplace letters. During the same period his adoptive-mother described him as increasingly dependent. On admission to hospital the only abnormal physical finding was a peculiar movement of the right arm which was considered to be a tic. The provisional diagnosis was a neurosis with regressive features. The initial EEG record was inconclusive, a repetitive pattern being interpreted as an artefact produced by the arm movement. It emerged that the patient had had a very unhappy childhood; his mother died when he was very young, and he was placed in a succession of foster-families, before finding a stable adoptive home. During the first fortnight in hospital delusions developed, a tentative diagnosis of schizophrenia made, and insulin therapy started. The first injection of insulin resulted in long-lasting coma during which the 'tic' was seen to be a stereotypy. By now the EEG record showed an unmistakable repetitive pattern typical of subacute sclerotizing pan-encephalitis.

CHRONIC CEREBRAL SYNDROMES

Cerebral palsy is present from birth, though the diagnosis may be delayed because techniques of neurological examination of the infant are difficult, and not yet widely known.

Organic impairment of the brain occurring later in life may be due to metabolic abnormalities which become clinically obvious only months or years after birth. Lesions resulting from the abnormal copper metabolism of Wilson's disease may result in damage to both liver and brain, affecting especially the basal ganglia. At the time of onset psychiatric features may predominate. Ingestion of lead, especially in children of poor families may cause a chronic encephalopathy.

In later childhood the demyelinating diseases may occasionally cause diagnostic difficulty. Subacute sclerotising encephalitis is probably caused by the measles virus. Schilder's disease may be present as hemianopsia followed by cortical blindness, though motor impairment may appear first. Multiple sclerosis is seen rarely in childhood but may also present initially with psychological symptoms.

The presence of a chronic brain syndrome calls for a full clinical evaluation, as follows:

1. The degree of *motor impairment*, e.g. muscle tone and power, balance, and coordination.

2. The presence of any *sensory handicap*, e.g. visual or auditory impairment following rubella infection, visual impairment resulting from congenital toxoplasmosis, perceptual deafness due to kernicterus.

3. *Intellectual status*. This may be very difficult to evaluate in the presence of sensory handicap. Special test procedures are available but require of the psychologist much experience in their administration. Specific learning difficulties affecting reading, writing, or arithmetic may be present.

4. *Convulsive tendency*. Where a brain syndrome and associated epilepsy are the result or organic damage the convulsions are usually much more resistent to anticonvulsant therapy than in the so-called idiopathic variety.

5. *Psychiatric assessment* aims at discovering the influence of the organic disorder on personality development, whether handicap or other limitation is accepted realistically, is denied, or leads to passive acceptance and dependency.

The term *minimal brain damage* (Strauss and Lehtinen, 1947) was intended to identify a syndrome of overactivity, distractability, and impulsiveness often associated with crossed-laterality but with indefinite or absent neurological signs. It is by no means certain that there is such a unique syndrome. There are, moreover, striking dissimilarities in epidemiology between otherwise comparable countries. For example Wender, (1971) on the basis of several studies estimates that there are between five and ten per cent of hyperactive children in the USA, whereas Bax (1972) in a study of 1200 five-year-old children living in the Isle of Wight did not find a single case. It seems likely that this is a heterogeneous collection of children, some highly intelligent with a strong exploratory drive, others reacting with anxiety to environmental stress, still others displaying depressive features, signs of emotional deprivation, or even obscure forms of epilepsy. (Koupernik *et al*, 1974.)

The concept of *minimal brain dysfunction* (Walzer and Wolff, 1973) is hardly less confusing. The differentiation of 'minimal' abnormality from normality is entirely a subjective appraisal, and explanations based on the idea of disorder of arousal mechanisms in the reticular formation remain speculative.

EPILEPSIES

Infantile spasms or *hypsarrhythmia* occur in the young infant often around the age of 6 months, the presenting symptoms being flexor spasms. In these the infant flexes the trunk and neck and at the same time brings the flexed upper limbs toward the midline. The seizures do not last more than about 30 seconds and occur frequently. The term hypsarrhythmia really means 'mountainous arrhythmia' referring to the highly abnormal EEG pattern. Permanent damage with intellectual impairment is by far the most frequent outcome. Less commonly psychotic-like features predominate. Administration of ACTH does seem to control the seizures but it is doubtful whether it affects the long term prognosis.

Petit mal is a very clear-cut variety more or less confined to early childhood and characterized by 'absences' with minimal motor accompaniments. The characteristic EEG pattern is of three per second 'spike and wave' discharges. Petit mal responds in a very selective way to two types of drugs, trimethadione and ethosuccinimide. There would appear to be no direct correlation between petit mal, grand mal, and associated intellectual or behavioural impairment. Nevertheless there are two important issues which can modify behaviour, namely the side-effects of drugs used in treatment, and the impact of the child's disorder on parents and family.

Lennox encephalopathy may resemble petit mal but has an earlier age of onset, is characterized by less clear-cut but longer 'absences', does not show the typical EEG patterns, and is unresponsive to compounds which control classical petit mal. The main difference, however, is that in this disorder there is progressive intellectual deterioration.

Grand mal is the most typical and the most impressive variety of epilepsy, the traditional 'falling sickness'. The attacks display a characteristic sequence in which loss of consciousness is succeeded by tonic spasms, and then by clonic jerks. Phenobarbitone, primidone, and hydantoin are the anticonvulsants of choice.

Seizures which are triggered by flickering light, for example from the television screen, are referred to as *photogenic epilepsy*.

Psychomotor or *temporal lobe epilepsy* from the clinical viewpoint is a very different entity. We should note first of all that in the majority of cases the condition is not related to an anatomically localized or focal lesion. The discharge can emanate from the centrencephalic medial structures and then follow a path through the temporal lobe. This explains the occasional modification of seizures in a child, generalized grand mal attacks later becoming focal fits. The first psychomotor attacks to be described were the uncinate olfactory fits (Hughlings Jackson). Other forms are visual, auditory or the more complex *praxic* or behavioural fits. The child may suddenly move the head and limbs, sometimes the whole body to one side, or replace normal activity by an abnormal and obviously unmotivated one. Psychomotor attacks are sometimes called *equivalents* and are not necessarily accompanied by loss of consciousness but by 'clouding'. Similar to these are the *dreamy states*, and experiences of *déjà vu*. There may be associated feelings of uneasiness or strangeness. A consistent feature is that the attacks are experienced as unpleasant, though occasionally they may be pleasurable with feelings of euphoria or even sexual orgasm.

From the prepubertal stage onwards psychomotor epilepsy may be accompanied by symptoms of anxiety and depression. The attacks are characteristically associated with feelings of strangeness. Such youngsters often have marked psychological problems of adjustment. The seizures may interfere with scholastic progress, and there may be resentment and lack of co-operation in taking anticonvulsant drugs. Sometimes it is difficult to disentangle the seizures themselves from associated hysterical behaviour. Occasionally psychotic episodes develop, often though not always in adolescence. The picture may closely resemble that of schizophrenia but here the EEG is abnormal with mainly unilateral or bilateral temporal foci.

Psychiatric disorder and epilepsy may be inter-related in a number of ways. Firstly, we may find a psychiatric illness such as a psychosis closely resembling schizophrenia caused directly by the organic impairment in the temporal part of the brain. Other psychological symptoms may be secondary to the fact of having the disorder, and of coping with the reactions of family, peers, and society. In order to understand the implications for a person of being epileptic it is useful to recall that during the Middle Ages the condition was regarded as evidence of diabolic possession. Even in recent times epilepsy continues to be considered by some as a stigma. It is frequently believed to be an hereditary disorder whereas in fact only a small percentage of epilepsies are genetic. This may lead to feelings of shame in the individual, and of guilt in the parents and family. There is still a tendency to segregate epileptic children at school and elsewhere. Nor has medical management always been wise in imposing excessive restriction of ordinary activities such as swimming, boating, and bicycling, all of which may be reasonable so long as there is adequate supervision. There is in fact no reason at all why a child or adolescent who is well-controlled on anticonvulsants should not attend a normal school. Families, however, frequently need a good deal of advice, support and, at times, psychiatric help in coping with the various problems as they arise.

Of some importance are the side effects of some anticonvulsant drugs. We are concerned here primarily with psychological effects but have to bear in mind that some of these medications can lead to blood dyscrasias and skin disorders. Children taking barbiturates, hydantoin or succinimide may become drowsy, and this can impair concentration. The drug dosage may then require to be reduced or combined with a stimulant such as amphetamine. The latter drug is probably also capable of preventing psychomotor seizures by maintaining the state of arousal. Nevertheless, because of the danger of addiction amphetamines should be prescribed very sparingly. Paradoxical drug effects are common in childhood. For instance as we have already noted amphetamines may have a sedative effect on hyperkinetic states, whereas the barbiturates may create a state of irritability.

We should notice finally that a child or more especially an adolescent may be unable to come to terms with the fact of suffering from epilepsy, and this psychological denial is reflected in an ambivalent attitude towards the taking of anticonvulsant drugs. By 'acting-out' in this way the child makes his condition worse so that we are confronted with a vicious circle. He may not readily accept sensible advice to avoid late nights and alcohol. An over protective as well as a rejecting attitude on the part of the parents can both lead to inadequate supervision. For these and other reasons it is clear that the management of such cases calls for a combined medical and psychosocial approach.

MENTAL HANDICAP

It seems likely that there are two groups of mentally handicapped individuals. In a given population the intelligence follows a Gaussian distribution curve. The left sector represents children of average or just below average ability and in this group sociocultural and emotional factors probably predominate. The other group consists of those children with very low ability and here organic causes can usually be identified.

Here we wish to discuss some aspects of diagnosis and prognosis, first of all how to interpret the results of intelligence testing. While these tests are useful the results should always be viewed in the context of a clinical appraisal. Raw scores alone are inadequate for assessment purposes and must be complemented by a qualitative description of the sample of childhood behaviour. For instance some children have poor concentration or very short attention-span; others a limited range of facial mimicry. Account has to be taken of the child's level of reasoning and problem-solving along the lines established by the work of Piaget. Some children are wrongly considered to be mentally handicapped when in fact they have a lag in language development. Very anxious or inhibited children may seem unable to answer questions or carry out tasks though in fact the ability is there. In effect this means that psychological testing can contribute significantly to a differential diagnosis. A number of points deserve special consideration:

(a) Where a child has lived in an environment with very poor stimulation there is often delay in intellectual development. This applies of course particularly to children suffering from emotional deprivation but it may also occur where the child grows up in a family with poor intellectual status or where there has been much disruption of family life. Social and cultural deprivation both play a large part here. There is a statistically significant difference in the IQ levels of children belonging to families of low economic and cultural status compared with those in more privileged situations and this is not explicable merely as a consequence of genetic endowment.

(b) A child may give the impression of being mentally handicapped but in fact may be suffering from a psychiatric disorder. High levels of anxiety readily interfere with intellectual function.

(c) Autistic children give very inconsistent performances, some of them for example being very good on verbal tests with an extraordinary memory, and yet are unable to adjust to a new situation or to solve simple problems. Figurative language often defeats them completely. In contrast other children who have practically no speech are able to solve quite difficult mechanical problems and can calculate. In this category is the 'idiot savant', a severely retarded individual with an island of good or even exceptional ability.

The IQ level on its own can be a misleading guide as regards educability. Some children of near average ability are very difficult to educate because they are extremely withdrawn, uncommunicative or hyperactive. Sometimes when the child's family background is a sophisticated one, where communication tends to be verbal, the child gives a spurious IQ which has been artificially raised. Comprehensive developmental assessment of a child must take into account all these various parameters, motor development, co-ordination, sensory integrity, and emotional adjustment.

It is probably time that we gave up altogether the notion of 'educability' as such. Even very poorly endowed children can be helped to improve their ability in everyday tasks often to a surprising degree although abstract intellectual functioning may be beyond them. It is for this reason that all handicapped children in England are now the responsibility of the Ministry of Education and Science and are not as formerly divided into those who are 'educable' and those who are not. A great difficulty is that although special workshops are now commonly provided both in the community and in hospital there is less and less opportunity for unskilled work in modern society. It is probably true also that in more primitive societies and even in rural communities there is a better acceptance and tolerance for the mentally handicapped than in the cities.

Often the presence of a handicapped child is extremely stressful for the family, leading to quite inappropriate focussing on the needs of the child to the detriment of the others. Sometimes there is marked overprotection, and failure to allow the child to progress even at his own rate. Outright rejection of such children is probably rather uncommon, but instances are known where such a child has been killed by the parents.

Mentally retarded individuals now live much longer than they did formerly, especially since the introduction of antibiotics. It is important, therefore, that everything possible should be done to give them a reasonable mode of life and as much independence as they can achieve. A great deal of experiment is going on in many parts of the world to move away from the traditional mental deficiency hospital or colony to smaller family-size units or hostels which are more closely related to the general community. We do not even know at the present time to what extent institutionalization of the handicapped has been responsible for many of the syndromes of slow development and behavioural disturbance which have formerly been regarded as an intrinsic part of mental handicap itself.

Prevention is within our scope in a number of fields. Good care of the expectant mother and expert obstetric supervision can reduce the incidence of damage to the foetus and newborn. It is possible to diagnose antenatally the presence of a number of chromosomal abnormalities or with the help of serological procedures the presence of active rubella infection. When abnormalities of this kind are detected or a high risk is estimated there are now ethical grounds for recommending termination of pregnancy. It is also possible now to detect carriers of a recessive disorder such as phenylketonuria. Finally with early diagnosis of this and related metabolic disorders the use of specialized diets from infancy onwards can prevent the development of mental retardation.

REFERENCES

Bax, M. (1972) (Personal Communication).

Koupernik, C., MacKeith, R., & Francis-Williams, J.H. (1975) Neurological correlates of motor and perceptual development. In *Perceptual and Learning Disabilities in Children.* vol 2. pp. 105–136. *Research and Theory.* Ed. Cruickshank, W.M. and Hallahan. C.P. Syracuse: Syracuse University Press.

Rutter, M., Graham, P. and Yule, W. (1970). A neuropsychiatric study in childhood. *London Clinics in Developmental Medicine,* 35/36.

Walzer, S. & Wolff, P.H. (eds.) (1973) Minimal Cerebral Dysfunction in Children, New York and London. Grune and Stratton.

Wender R.H. (1971) *Minimal Brain Dysfunction in Children.* New York: Wiley.

FURTHER READING

Ford, F.R. (1966) *Diseases of the Nervous System in Infancy, Childhood, and Adolescence,* 5th edn. Springfield, Ill.: Thomas.

Pond, D.A. (1965) The neuropsychiatry of childhood. In *Modern Perspectives in Child Psychiatry.* ed. Howells, J.G. Edinburgh: Oliver & Boyd.

MacKeith, R. and Bax, M. (eds.) (1963) Minimal cerebral dysfunction. *Clinics in Developmental Medicine.* 10.

Ounsted, C., Lindsay, J. and Norman, R. (1966) Biological factors in temporal lobe epilepsy. *Clinics in Developmental Medicine,* 22.

11

Treatment procedures

AIMS AND METHODS OF TREATMENT

The relief of stress

In the majority of cases there is likely to have been a considerable period of concern or even distress prior to actually seeking professional help. Whether this stems primarily from the child, parents, teacher, or someone else, relief is often first obtained by sharing the distress with one who is seen to be both concerned and competent. While concern by itself aids the expression of pent-up feeling, it is self-defeating unless backed by professional competence, and this is put to the first real test when the stage is reached, after initial assessment procedures have been completed, of giving an authoritative opinion. Most psychiatrists, and psychotherapists tend to be sceptical about the efficacy of reassurance and advice as generally understood, namely the assertion that there is nothing to worry about, because the expert says so. Even if the disorder is judged to be relatively minor, saying so gives at best temporary relief. The distress remains or returns unless reassurance is preceded by what is termed the 'working through' process. This means that time is made available in which sufficient trust is established to permit the airing of anxiety, and often guilt, sometimes rational but often with irrational components. Like patients seeking psychotherapeutic help in their own right parents come seeking advice. They expect to be told where they have gone wrong with their child or children, and how to put it right. That this is the correct and complete explanation of their problem may not even be questioned, though in some instances there is an underlying wish to be contradicted. Advice can be helpful, contrary to some traditional views, but must take its place as part of the 'working through' process, otherwise it will either not be heard, or more commonly will be misheard. The traditional medical approach in which a diagnostic explanation is followed by a provisional prognosis and a proposal regarding further therapeutic measures, if required, is an excellent guide in the context of child psychiatric practice, although as we have seen the term 'diagnosis' has a somewhat different connotation.

In many cases the help of the social worker will be required and the psychiatrist can do much to foster the case-work contact. It is important that the social worker be given a provisional outline of the assessment, a realistic clinical prognosis, and indication of the probable intrafamily dynamics, and some guidance regarding the kind of help the parents are likely to be able to use. This provides the social worker with guide-lines along which to proceed.

In many situations relief is affected only by direct intervention. Sometimes the symptom itself dictates the course of events, as for example, when an older child is suspected of suicidal preoccupations, or a younger boy or girl persistently engages in activities which endanger his or her own life. Such a patient requires, at least temporarily, to be in a place of safety. This may be a hospital psychiatric unit or a residential children's home or hostel, depending on local facilities. Running-away children pose similar problems regarding safety, as do some persistent truants. Hospitalization may also be indicated where there is uncontrollable aggression towards others, or sudden personality change, and especially if psychotic-like features are detected; or where persistent anorexia is accompanied by progressive weight loss.

The development of psychiatric *day-units* exclusively for children or adolescents has made it possible to manage many acutely presenting problems without the necessity of removing the child from home. Day-centre facilities for the young children, along with their parents if necessary ('therapeutic nurseries'), provide for the management of, for example, severe separation-anxiety precipitated by the attempted introduction of the child to nursery or school; for the overactive, distractible child excluded from school or nursery as a disruptive influence, and for the acute feeding or toileting problem which is so often a reflection of a disturbed mother-child relationship. An initial period of in-patient or day-care is often useful in the management of 'school refusal'.

The first consideration in all these instances is the relief of stress whether of the child, the parents, the teacher or the community. We can then proceed at a measured and controllable pace to explore further therapeutic possibilities.

'Stress-tolerance' varies enormously from one family to another, and indeed at different times in the same family, so that once again it is necessary to consider the child within his environment. Not only parents but teachers also may show great variation in their capacity to accept deviant behaviour or learning patterns, and crises may call for emergency relief. In some parts of Britain day schools for maladjusted children are used in this way.

Treatment procedures with the child

We have already described in some detail the technical aspects of the psychiatric interview with children. As we have seen this demands the ability to 'tune in' to the child's developmental level as regards language, comprehension, need for physical contact, as well as a sensitive awareness of non-verbal cues, the recognition of and ability to accept all variations of affect, and an understanding of the often obscure communications of the child's drawings, paintings, models and 'games'. It is a common experience that a first contact may be dominated by fear, defensiveness, and lack of trust so that several interviews are needed for any sort of assessment. It is also true that the first contact may be extremely revealing, that the unusually high level of anxiety may lower defences, permitting an immediate entrée to the child's inner world of suppressed feeling and thought, to private phantasy, or even occasionally to ordinarily deeply repressed material. Not only is it artificial, therefore, to designate an exploratory session as either 'diagnostic' or 'psychotherapeutic', but a first interview of the type described often provides a therapeutic opportunity which may not readily present itself during many subsequent contacts.

Psychotherapy with children is often conducted on a weekly basis, each session lasting up to an hour depending on the patient's age, developmental level, and emotional state. It is a common practice for the parents to be interviewed at the same time by the social work member of the clinical team (collateral therapy). For pre-school children, and even some older ones, play-materials provide the appropriate means of communication in addition to language. Painting, modelling, puppetry can all assist in gaining access to the imagination of young children. Face-to-face interviews begin to be useful and acceptable for many six or seven year olds, sometimes interspersed with play activity.

For selected children and adolescents, group therapy is useful and economical. For the younger ages, group play-psychotherapy, besides affording an excellent observation setting often provides an oppor-tunity to 'work-through' peer group difficulties, excessive fears and inhibitions with the support of the therapist. For older children the content of group-activity is modified appropriately. Many adolescents are able to participate in more formal group-discussion; some are candidates for psycho-drama, a technique of using spontaneous drama presentations for therapeutic ends.

Psycho-analysis is indicated for selected children with severe neurotic or personality problems. As this involves four or five clinic attendances per week it is not a practical proposition on a community scale.

Paradoxically there are certain circumstances in which it is important to allow a child to have symptoms in the knowledge that they are the expression of an emotional upheaval which, handled rightly, will be temporary. A child may display emotional regression after the birth of a sibling, following a separation experience (in the younger age-groups), or as part of a bereavement reaction. In these situations the re-appearance of dependency, separation-fears, wetting, or soiling is common but usually transient, provided they are handled sympathetically. Very similar regressive behaviour often accompanies a physical illness. Regression also occurs during certain critical phases of psychotherapy when the appearance of 'symptoms' may be an indication of progress.

Behaviour therapy with children is a recent development. Based on learning therapy, this is a direct approach on symptoms, in contrast to exploratory or depth psychotherapy which aims to uncover underlying attitudes, feelings, and wishes. In one respect the approaches are similar, namely the need for a warm, accepting, sensitive and enthusiastic approach by the therapist. Behaviour therapy seems to be most successful when the problem is monosymptomatic or at least circumscribed, for example in the treatment of a specific phobia. The use of the 'pad and bell' apparatus for nocturnal enuresis, which with a cooperative and motivated child has proved very successful, is an example of conditioning though the exact mechanism is unclear. 'Behaviour shaping', based on a reward system, has proved valuable in modifying dangerous or undesirable activities even in mentally handicapped children, for example where self-mutilation or self-induced vomiting have become established action patterns. A further approach is the use of the child's parents or teachers as therapists, by carrying out carefully prepared programmes at home or in school.

Remedial education may be undertaken by the educational psychologist or teacher. The aim here is to combine teaching with emotional support, and in the case of specific handicaps to employ specialised pedagogic techniques. Emotional release, a necessary prerequisite to learning in many cases, may be encouraged by the use of play, painting, story-writing and so on, though the actual medium is less important than the quality of rapport.

Chemotherapy. While the use of psychotropic drugs has been of major importance in the treatment of adult and to some extent adolescent patients, their application has been of less benefit to children. Medication amounts at best to symptomatic relief, and although this may sometimes be useful, drugs should not be used as a substitute for other treatment approaches. Many of the drugs to be considered produce unpleasant side-effects, which may be detrimental to physical growth and development. Moreover children may become habituated as readily as adults. The main groups of psychotropic durgs are:

1. Hypnotics
2. Sedatives
3. Tranquillizers
4. Anti-depressants
5. Stimulants

1. *Hypnotics.* These medications are used primarily to induce sleep. Insomnia is a common problem in children, especially the very young, and often has an emotional basis. Treatment therefore should be directed at the cause, but may be aided by the temporary administration of safe preparations such as triclofos a tasteless chloral derivative, or promethazine, an antihistamine with hypnotic properties. Nitrazepam is useful for older children and adolescents. Phenobarbitone is not recommended for children, except as an anticonvulsant, as it often excites rather than sedates.

2. *Sedatives.* A minor tranquillizer is sometimes useful in calming an anxious child during a short-term stressful experience. The safest and most useful drug is probably diazepam (which is also effective given parenterally in the management of status epilepticus). Diazepam and other benzodiazepines act by relaxing muscle tension and by central sedation, so that prolonged administration has a considerable risk of dependency for chronically anxious children and adolescents.

3. *Tranquillizers.* Chlorpromazine, the first of the phenothiazines to be introduced, is still the most effective drug in the treatment of schizophrenia and manic excitement in adults. It is equally effective in schizophrenic illness which occasionally begins in late childhood or adolescence, or for the emergency treatment of acute agitation and restlessness. In sunny weather thioridazine is preferable being less likely to produce skin sensitivity. The recently introduced butyrophenones (e.g. haloperidol) are probably equally effective and have fewer side-effects. Haloperidol has proved very effective in the treatment of tics.

The phenothiazines may have toxic effects on the bone-marrow, the liver, or the extra-pyramidal system. When prescribed in other than small doses, therefore, besides keeping the patient under regular review, an anti-Parkinsonian preparation should be administered jointly. To date, drugs have had no curative effect on the autistic disorders of early childhood (see Chapter 9).

4. *Anti-depressants.* These are of two main groups (a) tricyclics and (b) mono-amine oxidase inhibitors. The tricyclic anti-depressants are

primarily indicated in adults for endogenous depression, but this form of illness rarely appears in the pre-pubertal child. For the temporary symptomatic relief of a reactive depression in childhood imipramine is a relatively safe drug though there may be atropine-like side-effects such as dryness of the mouth and constipation. They are however potentially dangerous if taken in overdose. Imipramine and others in this group have been used with some success in the treatment of nocturnal enuresis, though the mode of action is unclear.

There is probably little justification for prescribing MAO inhibitors as the ingestion of foodstuffs containing tyramine e.g. cheese, yeast extracts, tinned fish may lead to a hypertensive crisis. Adrenaline, amphetamine, and imipramine are also incompatible.
5. *Stimulants.* As has been mentioned in Chapter 7 good results have been reported in hyperkinetic children by giving stimulants such as dextroamphetamine or methylphenidate. Why stimulants should paradoxically improve concentration and attention is by no means clear. Results, however, are not consistent, and a tranquillizer such as haloperidol may be more effective.

Modification of the environment.
Usually it will be found advisable, often essential, for the child's sessions to be paralleled by regular interviews with one or both parents. The parent therapist (psychiatrist or social worker) seeks to modify parental attitudes, often unconsciously determined, to act as an intermediary between child-therapist and parent, and to sustain the motivation for continuing attendance during phases of negative attitude by child, parents or both (*resistance*). This therapy programme involving parallel procedures for the child and parents is termed *collateral therapy.* Various modifications of this procedure may be used in special circumstances. Some therapists prefer to bring selected parents together in small groups of mothers, fathers or couples. *Conjoint family therapy* is a technique in which the therapy sessions include the parents, child, brothers and sisters. It is necessary to ensure that the marital situation is basically sound, and that neither parent suffers from a latent psychosis. The best results with this type of therapy are probably obtained where there is distortion or failure of communication between family members, especially a collusive silence regarding a too painful or threatening topic.

For every family which has sufficient inner resources and flexibility to benefit from psychotherapeutic intervention, we encounter many more which have not. Parental attitudes unconducive to healthy emotional development of children may be unmodifiable to any significant degree whether as a result of character disorder, deviant personality, severe psychoneurosis or a borderline psychotic state. Where this is so we may judge that the child has nevertheless sufficient personality resources to continue to develop reasonably satisfactorily, sometimes with an extended supportive contact; in others we may deem it imperative to remove the child to a different environment. By the time such a decision is reached, and an appropriate placement is found, the child will often for a variable period therefore require skilled handling based on a sensitive understanding of his own particular needs. Thus in recent years training courses have been developed in many countries to prepare carefully selected residential child-care staff for this exacting work. Increasing demands are being made on children's psychiatrists and their staffs to provide counselling services to such personnel.

Children suffering from severe and chronic illness with somatic, psychic and social components such as asthma, epilepsy and so on, in which family relationship patterns are playing a significant causal role, often present a particularly difficult problem of management because they may need both medical and psychiatric supervision, and for a variable period of time a substitute home. Specialized paediatric units and residential schools which meet both these requirements are gradually being developed in many countries.

Support

Though much of what applies here overlaps with the procedures previously described, we consider it important to discuss the supportive role in some detail. Firstly because in many instances it is the only helping role which is both appropriate and possible; and secondly because the concept of support has been denigrated by the implication that goodwill and perseverance alone are required. Workers in the mental-health field know only too well that a considerable proportion of their clients (a wider category than patients) given a supportive contact, though briefly and at quite long intervals, can function reasonably effectively between times, but rapidly deteriorate to ineffectuality, inappropriate behaviour or manifest mental illness if this prop is withdrawn. Where families with growing children are concerned this supportive role is undertaken by doctors, teachers, ministers of religion, community social workers, and not rarely by relatives and friends.

Let us consider, for example, the situation where the diagnosis is unequivocally that of a severely mentally handicapped child. In one instance where it is in the interests of the child and the family that care be maintained in the home it is often necessary to support the parents during the period of adjustment to the realities of the situation, as they pass from a phase of denial, of apparent acceptance, often to a kind of mourning grief, and gradually to a more balanced and realistic adjustment. Providing support at this crucial stage may be arduous, especially as irrational attitudes are frequently encountered. Advice about practical problems of management now begins to be 'heard'. In another family with a similarly affected child it may clearly be in the interests of the family as a whole that, at a particular age, a suitable long-term residential unit or home be found, but the parents resolutely oppose the recommendation. Here again skilled and often protracted support is required to help them overcome the sense of guilt that parting may entail. These same principles of aiding parental adjustment apply whenever a child is handicapped in some respect. The supportive technique which is appropriate to a given situation has to be based on an understanding of the psychic defence mechanism whereby a particular family copes. Seemingly inappropriate attitudes can then be understood, providing a rational basis for their modification.

Support is often a long-term undertaking especially when a child is suffering from deviant personality development such as autism or a complex developmental disorder such as hyperkinesis or *dysphasia*, and can only really be effective when combined with detailed knowledge of the clinical condition. Support may also be called for at times of family crisis due to illness, an abnormal birth, or bereavement, and recent investigations have shown that here also short-term help (*crisis intervention*) can be particularly effective in preventing long-term sequelae.

Promotion of mental health
As in every field of medical practice early treatment is preferable to late, and prevention is the ideal.

Child psychiatry has reached a phase of real dilemma inasmuch as wherever facilities for diagnosis and treatment have been developed the demand far outweighs the supply. It is doubtful whether in fact services can ever be adequate, as there can be no hard and fast criteria for what constitutes a severe enough problem to demand action. Even the fact that the patient is a young child does not guarantee that the disorder is mild or even curable. Nevertheless early detection of emotional difficulties is desirable, and general principles of management of the less severe understood by all those who care for children and adolescents. It is essential therefore that due emphasis be given to the principles of child-rearing, emotional development, and human relations in the training of doctors, nurses, and teachers. 'Primary prevention', that is the elimination of known pathogenic factors is as yet only realizable to a modest degree, and progress must await the results of research, still in a very early stage. Yet, even if our information is still imprecise, enough is already known about aetiological trends to indicate possible lines of action. Those employed in perinatal work are in a strategic position not only to minimize brain damage but also to detect the warning signs of unhealthy parental attitudes. Much can be done to avoid repeated or prolonged separation of young children from their parents. During the hospitalization of parent or child, contact can often be maintained by liberal visiting arrangements. Wherever cruelty or neglect is detected—and doctors are often in a key position so to do—this is likely to be a social case-work or even a psychiatric assignment.

In many countries much thought has already been given to the selection of adoptive parents, yet fostering tends to be a haphazard affair. Parent education programmes are enthusiastically promoted, attempts are made to reach prospective parents by provision for older school-children of courses in preparation for marriage, and inquiries have started into the problem of parental mental illnesses and its effects on children.

FURTHER READING

Freud, A. (1948) *The Psycho-analytic Treatment of Children*. London: Imago.

Caplan, G. (1961) *Prevention of Mental Disorders in Children*. New York: Basic Books.

Ginot, H.G. (1961) *Group Therapy of Children*. London: McGraw-Hill.

Koupernik, C. (1972) Chemotherapy in child psychiatry. *British Medical Journal* iii, 345–346.

Rutter, M. (1975) *Helping Troubled Children*. London: Penguin.

Skynner, A.C.R. (1969) A group-analytic approach to conjoint family therapy, *Journal of Child Psychology and Psychiatry*, 10, 81–106.

12

Child and family psychiatry

Throughout these preceding chapters we have tried to keep the child in his environmental and developmental perspective. We have sought always to take account of the child's stage and rate of development, as well as the quality of the setting in which he has his being. Nevertheless the model has been mainly a traditional medical one, the individual child as patient, the family or family substitute as the social setting which may influence development, contribute to the causation of disorder, and participate in therapeutic measures.

But the family is also a unit—which grows and develops, acquires a certain style, a set of values, attitudes towards other families, which may or may not be nourished by the community of which it is part, and in turn may contribute to a greater or lesser degree to the life of that larger community. It is within this living social organism that the children grow; when that growth is stunted or distorted it may be that we should seek causes also in the family unit itself.

We have already noted the emotional vulnerability of some children due to causes which may be genetically transmitted, or acquired early on as congenital factors; which may be due to organic brain pathology, or to early and severe emotional distortion or deprivation. Families may also be 'at risk' as regards their own well-being, and that of their members. There is much evidence of the vulnerability of one-parent families whether this be due to illegitimacy, separation, divorce, or bereavement. Another group is 'at risk' because of longstanding physical or mental illness of one or both parents. Anything which leads to continuous emotional stress, and repeated disorganization of the family is particularly threatening to the developing child, whether the manifest problem be alcoholism, drug abuse, financial irresponsibility or inadequacy of a father or mother, and especially where marital discord persists. Although poverty may play a significant part, children can grow up strong and healthy in a poor family. Nevertheless there can be situations where a whole community or cluster of families is under constant threat of disintegration, and which tend to foster delinquency and crime. These are areas of severe deprivation, which can be found in rural settings, though more often in the slums or barren housing estates of large cities, which in turn attract to themselves the least adequate migrant individuals and families, whose children tend to lack material, cultural, and often educational opportunity. This is the prevalent setting of juvenile delinquency, though occasionally the individual child's physical or mental state may be a contributory factor. These are not problems which clinics and clinicians can hope to solve but we shall return later to the theme of prevention.

While considering this broader spectrum of community life, it is worth noting, firstly that as regards the prevalence of emotional disorder in childhood it has been estimated in England that between 5 and 15 per cent of children suffer from disorders of sufficient severity to require skilled help (Underwood Report, 1955; Rutter *et al.*, 1970). Secondly, as an index of family break-up the number of children being cared for by local authorities during an average week in 1972 in England was not less than 60 000; even allowing that two-thirds of these are short-term emergency placements, six in every thousand children outwith an ordinary family setting is a formidable figure.

It is remarkable how many 'problem families' do succeed in rearing children successfully. These families of no fixed abode, with irregular income, and often little settled routine probably owe their cohesion, to the personality resources of the mother, who holds its members together.

Numerous studies have confirmed the long-term disadvantages in terms of health, emotional adjustment and educational progress of the illegitimate child, but we should note the complexities of this situation. In the past in most European countries at any rate, the unmarried mother and her child tended to be an ostracized pair; usually the child was accepted as a member of the grandparents' or other relative's family, or failing this was fostered, adopted, or reared in a residential home. The mother who kept her child tended to be the least equipped psychologically so to do. An unsuccessful outcome may therefore be due to factors other than illegitimacy. Now that a more liberal view begins to prevail, it is increasingly possible for an unmarried mother to keep her child, obtain accommodation, continue to benefit from the emotional support of relatives and friends, and to retain her self-respect.

Further changes in social attitudes include the widespread use of oral contraceptives, and in some countries, the legalised termination of pregnancies on social as well as medical grounds. One outcome has been the marked reduction in the number of infants presented for adoption. Secondly, those children for whom adoptive families tend not to be found so readily, are those in the older age-groups, those of mixed race, or those handicapped mentally, physically, or cosmetically. Adoption agencies are, therefore, obliged to screen the applicants, and are faced with the daunting task of assessing the motivation of the prospective adopters, and the likelihood of their being successful in their parental roles. Given skilled counselling and casework support, desirable though not always provided for adoptive parents, surprisingly good adjustments have been achieved with children as old as nine or ten years. (Kadushin, 1970)

The question as to whether the adopted child is at a disadvantage psychologically, is not easily answered. The most encouraging information comes from follow-up studies by Hoopes *et al.*, (1970) in America, and Seglow *et al.*, (1972) in Britain. The majority of agency placements do seem to work out well. There is no reliable information about 'direct' or 'third-party' placements. How then do we explain the disproportionate number of adopted children attending child-guidance and child-psychiatric clinics? It may be that adoptive parents as well as teachers and family doctors are highly motivated to seek psychiatric help for an adopted child when problems arise. We must recognize, however, that if there are latent psychological weaknesses in a marital or family situation, these are likely to be aggravated by undertaking adoption. It is interesting to contrast the practice in the Soviet Union where the fact of the adoption is deliberately concealed from the individual, with that in Western European Countries and in the USA of informing the child from an early age.

Even in families which are cohesive, problems of interpersonal relationships may arise. A persistently *overprotective attitude* to children is unhealthy, commonly inducing states of phobia and anxiety, psychosomatic syndromes, and inappropriate patterns of placating behaviour towards the parents (Levy, 1943). Markedly inconsistent patterns of rearing, expectations for behaviour or achievement, and of limit-setting may induce erratic, inconsistent responses. This may encompass all the offspring, a global or diffuse disorder of parent-child relationship, or single out one particular child in the family—a 'focal' disorder. Some workers such as Ackerman (1958) have drawn attention to families in which one member is manipulated by all the others into the role of a 'scapegoat', and behaves accordingly. The former is likely to be a reflection of the marital relationship or of a personality problem in the parent, the latter a specific circumstance or attribute relating to one particular child. Adler stressed the child's position in the family, and there is some evidence that where for example there are three children, the eldest tends to be successful (a fact demonstrated much earlier by Galton), the youngest the best adjusted emotionally, and the middle one the most vulnerable psychologically. But family position by itself can hardly be a major factor, except in the case of very large, poor families where the children have been shown to be progressively disadvantaged in relation to their ordinal position (Richards, 1969). Subtle relationship problems may result from a parent personally identifying with one of their children, or identifying one child with some other adult such as grandparent, uncle or aunt. Such identifications, predominantly unconscious, are revealed by inconsistent or even irrational behaviour towards the child. These disturbances can be seen as an extension of parental neurosis, the more usual symptoms being replaced by distorted patterns of interaction with the child. The treatment is similar to that of a neurosis, but the focus is on the child and the family, rather than on the sufferer and his past. Almost invariably a three-generation pattern is revealed, parental patterns being related in varying ways to their own relationships, especially in childhood, with the grandparents.

Investigations into the causes of *child abuse*, and in particular 'the battered baby' (Helfer and Kempe, 1968) have demonstrated that while a minority of the offending parents are mentally ill, most are not, but display immature, impulsive personalities, and frequently have themselves had disorganized early lives, with experiences similar to those they re-enact with their children. Cruelty and deprivation may produce a wide range of childhood symptoms, generalized anxiety, slowing of intellectual development, physical stunting, insecure sphincter control of bowels and bladder, impaired capacity for making relationships, and anti-social behaviour. With such families, support and direction is a more realistic goal than insight-orientated case-work or psychotherapy. This group alone strains to the limit our community resources for family and child care. It is moreover in this type of family that incest tends to occur. This usually involves brother-sister, or father-daughter relationships, rarely mother-son. Serious psychiatric after-effects are most likely in girls involved in paternal incest. These are usually large working-class families, in poor living conditions, where the parents display marked personality disorders. It is difficult to isolate the one factor of incest from this whole constellation of social pathology. Children of incestuous union display a greater morbidity and mortality than average.

Major mental illness in a parent can also severely test family resilience, particularly where external supports are weak. This is but one of many situations where spontaneous informal help from relatives, friends, and neighbourhood group can be so effective. When any mentally ill parent is admitted to hospital enquiries should automatically be made about the welfare of the children, especially younger ones. This problem demonstrates the poor co-ordination of general psychiatry, child psychiatry, and child care facilities in many communities.

THE FAMILY WITH A HANDICAPPED CHILD

This topic calls for separate consideration because the fact of having a child handicapped by chronic ill-health, physical abnormality, mental retardation or deviant personality inevitably creates a situation of psychological stress. This in turn may have repercussions for the affected child, any or all of the members of the family. As a generalization we may say that chronic worry is in itself enervating. At one time superstition and fear combined to produce situations of shame and concealment, so that the backward or deformed child might be hidden from sight for long periods and sometimes exposed to cruelty and neglect. Such situations must now be rare, yet the attitudes to handicapped persons are still often ambivalent. Critical periods for such families are at birth, when the time approaches for beginning school, sometimes with the onset of puberty, and often at school-leaving age. At all such stages professional help may be needed, in particular skilled counselling, and often the family doctor is best placed to undertake this task. He often has to deal with sheer reluctance to face the issues, with irrational guilt about aetiology, or with denial of the handicap itself. Some families adjust remarkably well to the special situation, a few disintegrate, while others focus excessively on the handicapped child to the relative neglect of the family as a whole. Parental rejection of such a child is rather rare; overprotection is common. Specialists in particular medical fields, such as paediatrics, mental deficiency, orthopaedics, and so on may contribute significantly at given times but the essential supportive role to the parents and the family requires a long-term, personalized contact. Lindemann (1944), and Caplan (1964) show how effective can be short-term psychological aid at times of major crisis, so-called *crisis intervention* technique. It is important also that we do not get out of perspective the present-day emphasis on 'community care'. It is true that many handicapped persons including children would be better living with their families, supported by day-centre provision, or in part-time residential hostels near their homes, but for some families and indeed for some handicapped persons such arrangements would create excessive burdens for either or both.

FAMILY DIAGNOSIS AND FAMILY THERAPY

Child psychiatric practice has always tended to view the patient in the context of family and community. Neither an exclusively child-centred nor parent-centred approach is adequate in diagnosis, treatment or prognosis. Too often, however, it is the mother and child only who attend child psychiatric or child guidance clinic, even when it is known that the family as a whole is involved in the problem. Traditionally the method of viewing the whole family was by home visiting, usually by a social-worker. Some centres invite the whole family to attend intake sessions. We have been alerted in recent years to the child 'patient' who is in fact the symptom of a 'sick' family. We have learned to recognize the mutually dependent family whose members, confronted by a threat to the security of the group (e.g. unemployment, illness, bereavement), all develop stress symptoms e.g. the father's peptic ulcer gives trouble again, the mother has a recurrence of migraine, one child starts complaining of abdominal pain, another reverts to bed-wetting; even the baby goes 'off colour' and may start vomiting. Here the family is 'the patient'—not at all a difficult concept for family doctors.

Family group therapy consists of regular interviews by the therapist of the parents and children together, and seems to be particularly helpful where the main difficulty is one of adequate communication between the members, especially where emotionally charged material such as grief, rage and guilt is not shared. A main aim of family group therapy is the sharing of such charged material. Depending on the intellectual level, and the degree of sophistication of the family, techniques may range from interpretation of hidden or unconscious motives, to the statement of avoided feeling coupled with support. The acquisition of such therapeutic skills demands sensitivity, resilience, and a capacity for honest self-regard. Balint (1961) has pioneered the training of general practitioners in this and related fields. New facilities are being developed to provide suitable psychiatric accommodation for total families requiring treatment. For this there is encouraging precedent in the work of *Family Service Units* in Britain who have dealt in a pragmatic way with socially and psychologically inadequate families. Bateson (1956), Laing (1960), Lidz (1964) and others have drawn attention to distorted relationships and communications commonly presented in the families of schizophrenics. It is by no means proven, however, that such inter-personal distortions are the root causes of schizophrenia, nor that their modification leads to cure.

One of our aims throughout this book has been to emphasize the multifactorial causation of childhood emotional disorders. Prevention requires to be undertaken on a broad front, where the psychiatrist takes his place alongside medical colleagues in many fields, with the psychologist and the social worker. To safeguard the emotional well-being of families and the development of their children involves us in standards of antenatal, natal, and postnatal care, availability of genetic counselling, and the education of medical students and doctors in the emotional needs of childhood and adolescence.

REFERENCES

Ackerman, N.W. (1958) *The Psychodynamics of Family Life* New York: Barie Books.

Bateson, G. (1956) Toward a theory of schizophrenia. *Behavioural Science*, 1, 251.

Hoopes, J.L. (1970) *A Follow-up Study of Adoptions*. Child Welfare League of America.

Kadushin, A. (1970) *Adopting Older Children* New York: Columbia University Press.

Laing, R.D. (1960) *The Divided Self*. London: Tavistock.

Levy, D.M. (1943) *Maternal Overprotection*. New York. Columbia University Press.

Lidz, T. (1964) *The Family and Human Adaptation*. London: Hogarth.

Lindemann, E. (1944) Symptoms and management of acute grief. *American Journal of Psychiatry*, 101.

Richards, I.D. (1969) Perinatal Mortality in Glasgow Health Bulletin, XXVII, 4.

Rutter, M., Tizard, J., & Whitmore, K. (1970) *Education, Health and Behaviour*, Edinburgh: Longman.

Seglow, J., Kellmer Pringle M., & Wedge, P. (1972) *Growing Up Adopted*. London: National Foundation for Education Research.

FURTHER READING

Association of British Adoption and Fostering Agencies (1977) *Child Adoption*. London.

Balint, M. & Balint, E. (1961) *Psychotherapeutic Techniques in Medicine*. London: Tavistock.

Gould, J. (ed.) (1968) *The Prevention of Damaging Stress in Children*. London: Churchill.

Helfer, R.E. & Kempe, C.H. (ed.) (1968) *The Battered Baby*. Chicago: Univ. of Chicago Press.

Hunt, P. (ed.) (1966) *Stigma. The Experience of Disability*. London: Chapman.

Stone, F.H. (1976) *Psychiatry and the Paediatrician*. London: Butterworths.

Underwood Report of Committee on Maladjusted Children (1955) London: HMSO.

Glossary

Acting out
Difficult, often disruptive behaviour in response to unresolved conflicts or anxieties. Derived originally from 'acting-out of transference'.

Affectionless character
Abnormal childhood personality characterized by impairment in development of conscience and capacity to form lasting interpersonal relationships. (Bowlby)

Ambivalence
Attitude towards a person or situation containing both positive and negative elements.

Attachment
syn. **Bonding**. Describes the earliest stages of the reciprocal relationship between mother and infant.

Bonding
See **Attachment**.

Conduct disorder
Heterogeneous group of behaviour disturbances, giving rise to social disapproval; more common in boys.

Conflict (intrapsychic)
State of emotional unease due to the presence of deeply felt but opposing wishes or drives; may become 'buried' or unconscious.

Conversion hysteria
Bodily dysfunction e.g. deafness, paresis, anaesthesia symptomatic of hysterical disorder. Name derived from explanation that repressed libidinal energy is converted into bodily symptom.

Counter-transference
Converse of transference i.e. irrational attitude of therapist towards patient, displaced from significant person in therapist's present or past life situation.

Defences
syn. **Defence Mechanisms**. Psychological methods of coping with stress, especially unresolved conflicts. e.g. projection, identification, repression. May present as symptom e.g. counter-phobia.

Delinquency
Persistent anti-social behaviour in conflict with the law, short of criminality.

Dysphasia, congenital
Developmental language disorder. e.g. sensory dysphasia is a disturbance in the comprehension of the spoken word; expressive aphasia a disturbance of motor speech.

Dyspraxia
Disability in carrying out complex motor activities.

Echolalia
Echo-speech. Characteristic of speech of autistic children.

Encopresis
Faecal soiling, beyond the usual stage of sphincter control.

Enuresis   Persistent voiding of urine beyond the usual stage of sphincter control.

Folie à deux   Situation in which two persons, for example husband and wife or parent and child, share a delusional belief or attitude, initiated by one of them.

Hyperkinetic syndrome   Extreme, persistent pattern of over-activity usually seen in younger age groups and associated either with psychogenic disturbance or organic brain disorder.

Iatrogenic   lit. Caused by the physician; usually refers to unintentional complication of medical intervention.

Introjection   A psychological process postulated by psycho-analytic theory whereby a child internalizes the attitudes and values of the parents.

Kernicterus   Cerebral complication of hyperbilirubinaemia in the newborn, usually the outcome of rhesus incompatibility. May result in irreversable neurological damage, mainly of extrapyramidal system.

Narcissism   Intense self-love. In psychoanalytic theory an early stage of psycho-sexual development in which the child is the object of his own love, and which in an adult represents an extreme degree of emotional immaturity or regression.

Oedipus complex   Characteristic phase of normal psycho-sexual development usually during third to sixth years of age in which child is possessive of parent of opposite sex and in rivalry with parent of same sex.

Paranoid schizophrenia   The most frequently encountered form of this mental illness, characterised by delusional ideas of persecution. Not to be confused with a 'personality'; over suspicious but not delusional.

Parental over-protection   Over-solicitous attitude of parent towards child.

Phantasy   State of sustained imagination with either pleasurable or frightening content.

Phobia   Persistent irrational fear of object or situation. e.g. animal-phobia, agoraphobia.

Projection   Mental mechanism in which thoughts or attitudes are ascribed to someone else. Characteristic of paranoid states.

Projective tests   Psychological tests which attempt to elicit personality traits through stimuli such as pictures, ink-blots or sentences requiring completion.

Reality testing   The ability to distinguish reality from phantasy.

Regression   syn. **Emotional Regression**. Reappearance of behaviour and attitudes appropriate to a younger age level, often in response to situation of insecurity. e.g. child following a separation experience, in response to birth of sibling, during a physical illness.

Ritual   Repetitive, apparently purposeless activity, often quite complex, seen typically in obsessional neuroses and occasionally in psychoses, but also frequently a transient manifestation in young children.

Separation anxiety Distress manifested by child on separation or threat of separation from person to whom there is stong attachment, e.g. parent or parent substitute; normal manifestation of emotional development, maximal between two or three years.

Sibling rivalry Aggressive competitiveness with brother or sister; often immediately younger one in family, for affection of one or both parents.

Testing-out Repetitive challenge by child or adolescent to the authority of parent, teacher, etc.

Thought omnipotence Phantasy, usually of young children, that wishes or thoughts by themselves are sufficient to determine events. e.g. death-wishes.

Transference Characteristic phenomenon during psychoanalysis in which patient's feelings, attitude, behaviour towards therapist are in fact a displacement from a significant figure in the patient's present of past life; described as positive if feelings are affectionate, negative if hostile.

Index

CHURCHILL LIVINGSTONE MEDICAL TEXTS

**Tumours – Basic Principles and
Clinical Aspects**
Christopher Louis

The Essentials of Neuroanatomy
Third Edition
G. A. G. Mitchell and D. Mayor

Sexually Transmitted Diseases
Third Edition
C. B. S. Schofield

Notes on Medical Virology
Sixth Edition
Morag C. Timbury

Clinical Pharmacology
Third Edition
P. Turner and A. Richens

**Immunology: An Outline for Students
of Medicine and Biology**
Fourth Edition
D. M. Weir

LIVINGSTONE MEDICAL TEXTS

Geriatric Medicine for Students
J. C. Brocklehurst and T. Hanley

An Introduction to Clinical Rheumatology
William Carson Dick

Psysiology – A Clinical Approach
Second Edition
G. R. Kelman

A Concise Textbook of Gastroenterology
M. J. S. Langman

Introduction to Clinical Examination
Second Edition
Edited by John Macleod

Nutrition and its Disorders
Second Edition
Donald S. McLaren

An Introduction to Primary Medical Care
David Morrell

Urology and Renal Medicine
Second Edition
J. B. Newsam and J. J. B. Petrie

Psychological Medicine for Students
John Pollitt

Respiratory Medicine
Malcolm Schonell

An Introduction to General Pathology
W. G. Spector

Introduction to Clinical Endocrinology
John A. Thomson

Cardiology for Students
Max Zoob